SYNC YOUR CYCLE

SYNC YOUR CYCLE

HARNESS YOUR MENSTRUAL CYCLE FOR
HORMONAL HARMONY AND HOLISTIC WELLNESS

WOMEN'S HEALTH

LILA LACY

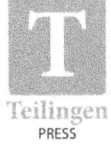

Teilingen
PRESS

Copyright © 2023 by Lila Lacy

All rights reserved. No part of this book may be reproduced, stored in a retrieval system, or transmitted in any form or by any means, electronic, mechanical, photocopying, recording, or otherwise, without the prior written permission of the publisher, Teilingen Press.

The information contained in this book is based on the author's personal experiences and research. While every effort has been made to ensure the accuracy of the information presented, the author and publisher cannot be held responsible for any errors or omissions.

This book is intended for general informational purposes only and is not a substitute for professional medical, legal, or financial advice. If you have specific questions about any medical, legal, or financial matters matters, you should consult with a qualified healthcare professional, attorney, or financial advisor.

Teilingen Press is not affiliated with any product or vendor mentioned in this book. The views expressed in this book are those of the author and do not necessarily reflect the views of Teilingen Press.

This book is dedicated to the women who have longed to dance in harmony with their own bodies. May this book be a beacon that guides you to the empowering shores of self-awareness and vibrant health. Embrace your cycle, embrace your power.

A woman's health is her capital.

— HARRIET BEECHER STOWE

CONTENTS

Embracing the Power of Your Cycle   xi

1. UNDERSTANDING YOUR MENSTRUAL CYCLE   1
   Hormones and Their Functions   3
   Tracking Your Cycle: Methods and Tools   6
   Common Myths and Misconceptions   7
   Chapter Summary   9

2. NUTRITION AND YOUR CYCLE   11
   Eating for Your Menstrual Phase   12
   Eating for Your Follicular Phase   13
   Eating for Your Ovulatory Phase   14
   Eating for Your Luteal Phase   16
   Supplements and Your Cycle   18
   Chapter Summary   19

3. EXERCISE AND YOUR CYCLE   21
   Adapting Workouts to Your Menstrual Phase   22
   Adapting Workouts to Your Follicular Phase   23
   Adapting Workouts to Your Ovulatory Phase   25
   Adapting Workouts to Your Luteal Phase   26
   Listening to Your Body: Signs and Signals   27
   Chapter Summary   29

4. CYCLE ALIGNMENT IN YOUR PERSONAL LIFE   31
   Social Engagements and Your Cycle   31
   Sex and Intimacy: Syncing with Your Partner   32
   Self-Care and Pampering Throughout the Cycle   34
   Emotional Well-being and Hormonal Fluctuations   35
   Planning Personal Events and Activities by Cycle Phase   37
   Chapter Summary   38

5. CYCLE ALIGNMENT IN YOUR PROFESSIONAL LIFE   41
   Productivity and Your Menstrual Cycle   41
   Communication and Collaboration During Different Phases   43
   Chapter Summary   44

6. **CYCLE ALIGNMENT AND FERTILITY** — 47
   - Natural Family Planning and Cycle Awareness — 48
   - Optimizing Fertility Through Lifestyle Choices — 50
   - Dealing with Infertility and Cycle Irregularities — 51
   - Preconception Care and Cycle Alignment — 53
   - Chapter Summary — 54

7. **CYCLE ALIGNMENT FOR HEALTH CONDITIONS** — 57
   - PCOS and Cycle Alignment — 57
   - Endometriosis and Menstrual Health — 58
   - Thyroid Health and Menstrual Regulation — 60
   - Managing PMS and PMDD with Cycle Awareness — 61
   - The Impact of Stress on Your Menstrual Cycle — 63
   - Chapter Summary — 64

8. **HOLISTIC APPROACHES TO CYCLE ALIGNMENT** — 67
   - Integrating Mindfulness and Meditation — 67
   - Herbal Remedies and Menstrual Health — 68
   - Acupuncture and Traditional Chinese Medicine — 70
   - Yoga and Cycle Syncing — 71
   - The Role of Sleep in Hormonal Balance — 73
   - Chapter Summary — 74

9. **CREATING YOUR PERSONAL CYCLE ALIGNMENT PLAN** — 77
   - Setting Goals and Intentions — 79
   - Designing Your Personalized Cycle Alignment Strategy — 80
   - Implementing and Adjusting Your Plan — 82
   - Tracking Progress and Making Data-Driven Decisions — 83
   - Chapter Summary — 85

10. **THE FUTURE OF CYCLE ALIGNMENT** — 87
    - The Role of Technology in Cycle Alignment — 88
    - Expanding the Conversation: Education and Advocacy — 90
    - Building a Community Around Menstrual Health — 91
    - Envisioning a Society in Sync with Cycles — 93
    - Chapter Summary — 95

    Your Journey Beyond the Pages — 97

    About the Author — 103

EMBRACING THE POWER OF YOUR CYCLE

Imagine if you could tap into a hidden superpower—one that ebbs and flows just like the tides, governed by the moon's pull. Your menstrual cycle holds this power, a rhythmic dance of hormones that, when understood and honored, can elevate your well-being to new heights. This isn't just about managing your period; it's about embracing the full spectrum of your cycle's phases, each with its own secret code to unlock your body's potential.

Think of your cycle as a symphony, with each movement expressing a different mood and energy. By tuning into this natural rhythm, you can live your life with more grace and vitality. It's about aligning your daily habits—from the food you savor to the movements you enjoy—with the natural flow of your body's menstrual cycle. There are numerous names for this process of alignment, including cycle syncing, cycle awareness, cycle optimization and hormone-based living.

Embracing the Power of Your Cycle

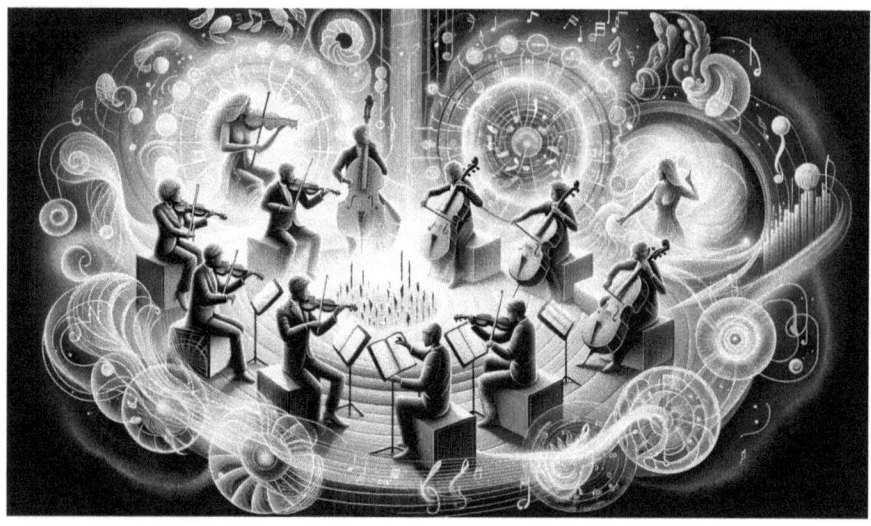

This journey into synchronizing your cycle is a path to empowerment. It's a call to listen intently to the whispers of your body and respond with nurturing care. As you learn to ride the waves of your hormonal shifts, you'll discover a profound connection with yourself that's both grounding and liberating.

The rewards of this alignment are as rich and varied as life itself. Women who embrace this wisdom often speak of a newfound zest for life, smoother cycles, and a clearer mind. It's a lifestyle that honors your body's innate wisdom, allowing you to move with the rhythms of nature rather than against them.

As we embark on this adventure together, we'll uncover the secrets of your cycle, transforming what you may have thought of as a monthly inconvenience into a source of strength and synchronization. You'll learn to make choices that resonate deeply with your body's needs, empowering you to live a life that's not just in sync with your cycle but also in tune with your truest self.

So, let's turn the page and begin this transformative journey. Your body is ready to reveal its secrets—are you ready to listen?

Self-Awareness and Body Wisdom

Step into the world of self-discovery, where the simple act of understanding your body becomes a radical act of self-care. In today's fast-paced society, we often become disconnected from the natural rhythms that govern our well-being. But imagine if you could reclaim that connection, tuning into the ebb and flow of your own biology with the finesse of a masterful conductor.

Your menstrual cycle is not just a biological process; it's a gateway to a deeper understanding of who you are. It's a monthly voyage that invites you to explore your body's inner workings, listen to its subtle cues, and respond with compassion and intelligence. This is where the magic happens—you begin to move in harmony with your intrinsic rhythms, and life unfolds more easily and synchronicity.

In embracing this dance of self-awareness, you're not just synchronizing your cycle; you're charting a course to a more empowered you. It's a journey that challenges the status quo and can help you live a life where your health and happiness are not left to chance but are consciously crafted with each phase of your cycle in mind.

This is about more than just surviving your menstrual cycle; it's about thriving within it. By becoming attuned to your body's signals, you unlock a wealth of knowledge that empowers you to make choices that support your physical, emotional, and mental health. It's an invitation to honor your body's natural wisdom, embrace its fluctuations, and celebrate its strength.

As we delve deeper into the art of aligning with your cycle, you'll find that this isn't just a practice; it's a reawakening. It's a call to reconnect with the most primal parts of yourself and to live a life that's not just balanced but vibrantly alive. So, take a deep breath and prepare to embark on a journey that will transform how you view your cycle, body, and potential.

Embracing the Power of Your Cycle

Charting the Course of This Book

As we begin this journey together, let's unfold the map that will guide us through the rich terrain of your cycle. We'll navigate through the valleys and peaks of your hormonal landscape, discovering treasures of wisdom at every turn.

First, we'll embark on an expedition to understand the phases of your menstrual cycle, demystifying the science and the soul of your monthly rhythm. You'll learn to recognize the landmarks of your hormonal journey and how to harness their power.

Then, we'll explore nutrition and its impact on your cycle, where the foods you eat can become allies and nourish you in sync with the shifting tides of your hormones. We'll cultivate a feast that satisfies your palate and supports your cycle's unique nutritional needs. Exercise becomes an expression of self-love, a way to celebrate and strengthen your body in alignment with your cycle's phases. We'll provide guidance that can help you find the rhythm of movement that resonates with the beat of your body.

We'll then weave the wisdom of your cycle into the tapestry of your personal and professional life. You'll learn how to schedule and go about your days with the colors of your inner cycle, creating a masterpiece of balance and productivity.

We'll also touch on fertility, the healing potential for health conditions, and holistic cycle alignment approaches.

Armed with this new knowledge, you'll become the master of your own cycle and develop the confidence to create your cycle alignment habits that align with your life's unique contours. And finally, we'll gaze into the horizon at the future of cycle alignment, envisioning a world where every woman's cycle is a source of strength and empowerment.

This book is your invitation to a grand adventure, a call to journey inward and emerge with a profound connection to the ebb and flow of your own body. So lace up your boots, dear explorer—the path to syncing with your cycle awaits, and the possibilities are as boundless as your own potential.

Embracing the Power of Your Cycle

Your Personal Odyssey: Navigating the Pages Ahead

As you stand at the start of this grand adventure, know that you are about to embark on a personal journey that promises to be as unique as you are. This book is not a one-size-fits-all manual but a treasure map to chart your course through the waters of cycle alignment.

Approach each chapter with curiosity and an open heart. You may choose to read this book from cover to cover, immersing yourself in the whole experience, or you may wish to navigate directly to the chapters that call out to you and resonate with the questions that bubble up from within you.

This is your adventure, and you are the captain. This book is a living document meant to be filled with your thoughts, reflections, and revelations. It is a space for you to converse with yourself, ask questions, and discover answers that are true to your soul.

And as you chart your journey, remember that this book is but one star in a constellation of resources. There may be companion guides, online communities, and workshops that serve as fellow travelers, offering support and camaraderie as you explore the wonders of your cycle.

So, take a deep breath, and prepare to embark on a journey of self-discovery that will transform not just how you view your cycle but how you live each day.

The future is a canvas stretched before you, and you hold the brush. Let the rhythm of your cycle be the stroke that guides you, painting a life that is as dynamic, beautiful, and profound as the journey you're about to undertake.

1

UNDERSTANDING YOUR MENSTRUAL CYCLE

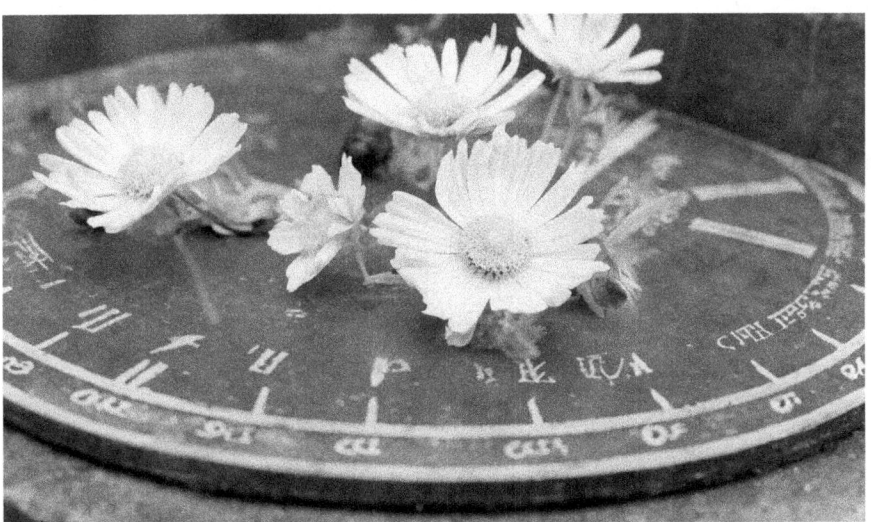

Embarking on the journey to understand your menstrual cycle is akin to unlocking a deeper level of self-awareness. The menstrual cycle is not just a biological process but a complex interplay of hormones that influence your physical health, emotional well-being, and overall lifestyle. To fully harness the power of your hormones and harmonize your daily habits with your cycle, it is essential first to understand the distinct phases of the menstrual cycle and the physiological changes they involve.

The menstrual cycle can be divided into four primary phases: the menstrual phase, the follicular phase, ovulation, and the luteal phase. Each phase is characterized by hormonal fluctuations and bodily responses that affect energy levels, mood, appetite, and overall well-being.

The menstrual phase marks the beginning of the cycle, where the lining of the uterus is shed if fertilization has not occurred. This phase is commonly known as your period and can last anywhere from a few days to a week. During this time, hormone levels, particularly estrogen and progesterone, are at their lowest, which can lead to the common symptoms of menstruation, such as cramps, fatigue, and mood swings. Many women report feeling more introspective and may benefit from gentle activities and nourishing foods during this time.

The follicular phase follows, and it typically culminates with the body preparing for ovulation. This phase can last about 7 to 10 days and is characterized by a rise in estrogen and follicle-stimulating hormone (FSH), which stimulates the growth of follicles in the ovaries and causes the uterine lining to thicken again in preparation for a potential pregnancy. This phase is often associated with increased energy, mental clarity, and creativity. Leveraging this time for brainstorming, planning, and engaging in more vigorous physical activities can be advantageous.

Ovulation is the pinnacle of the menstrual cycle, a brief but critical phase that usually occurs mid-cycle, around day 14 in a 28-day cycle. The surge in estrogen from the follicular phase leads to a spike in luteinizing hormone (LH), which triggers the release of an egg from the ovary into the fallopian tube. Estrogen peaks just before ovulation, and many women experience heightened senses, energy, and libido. This is when you are most fertile, and the body is primed for conception. Ovulation is often accompanied by physical signs such as a slight rise in basal body temperature and changes in cervical mucus. This phase can be an optimal time for socializing, high-intensity workouts, and critical decision-making.

Following ovulation, the ruptured follicle transforms into the corpus luteum, which secretes progesterone. Progesterone works in concert with estrogen to maintain the endometrial lining, creating a supportive environment for an embryo. If fertilization does not occur, the corpus luteum degenerates, leading to a drop in progesterone and estrogen levels. This hormonal shift causes the endometrial lining to shed, resulting in menstruation, and the cycle begins anew. During the luteal phase, some women may experience premenstrual symptoms. It's a period that may call for self-care, reflection, and preparation for the cycle to restart.

Understanding these phases and their hormonal changes is empowering. It allows for a deeper comprehension of your body's natural rhythms. By recognizing the ebb and flow of your hormonal landscape, you can tailor your nutrition, exercise, social life, and work tasks to harmonize with your body's flow. This alignment fosters a sense of harmony within and empowers you to make informed decisions that can enhance your productivity, vitality, energy, and wellbeing.

Cycle synchronization is not a one-size-fits-all approach; it's a personalized journey that evolves with you. It is about aligning with the body's natural state at any given time. It gives you the confidence to make informed choices that honor your body's needs, leading to a more balanced and fulfilled life.

Hormones and Their Functions

At the heart of cycle syncing is the endocrine system, which plays a pivotal role in regulating menstrual cycles. The endocrine system is a network of glands that secrete hormones directly into the bloodstream. These are all controlled by the hypothalamus, the brain's hormone control center. Your hormones, in turn, act as messengers, influencing various bodily functions, including reproduction, metabolism, and mood.

To truly understand and benefit from cycle alignment, we will explore the key hormones involved in your menstrual cycle, the functions they serve, and how their levels change throughout your cycle in more depth.

Estrogen

Estrogen is pivotal in the development of secondary sexual characteristics and the thickening of the uterine lining (endometrium) during the follicular phase in preparation for potential pregnancy. It also regulates the menstrual cycle and affects various other bodily systems.

Estrogen levels rise steadily during the follicular phase, peaking just before ovulation. After ovulation, levels drop sharply and rise slightly during the luteal phase before falling again before menstruation.

Progesterone

Progesterone is essential for maintaining the endometrium, which is necessary for the implantation of a fertilized egg and sustaining early pregnancy. It also helps regulate the menstrual cycle and affects mood and libido.

Progesterone levels remain low during the follicular phase and begin to rise after ovulation, reaching their peak in the middle of the luteal phase. If pregnancy does not occur, progesterone levels fall, leading to the shedding of the uterine lining and the start of menstruation.

Follicle-Stimulating Hormone (FSH)

FSH is crucial for the growth and maturation of ovarian follicles containing the eggs. It also stimulates the production of estrogen by the ovaries.

FSH levels increase at the beginning of the cycle, during the follicular phase, to stimulate follicle development. They peak early in the cycle and then decline as estrogen levels rise.

Luteinizing Hormone (LH)

LH triggers ovulation—the release of a mature egg from the ovary. It also stimulates progesterone production by the corpus luteum, the follicle remnant after the egg is released.

LH levels surge mid-cycle, leading to ovulation. This LH surge is brief but crucial for the release of the egg and the subsequent rise in progesterone during the luteal phase.

Testosterone

Although often considered a male hormone, testosterone is also present in females and plays a role in libido, bone health, and the maintenance of muscle mass. It can also influence mood and energy levels.

Testosterone levels are relatively constant but experience a slight increase around the time of ovulation, which can contribute to a rise in sexual desire during this phase of the cycle.

The interplay of all of these hormones is not only fundamental to reproductive health but also affects physical and emotional well-being. By tuning into these hormones and their fluctuations throughout your cycle, you can cultivate a sense of harmony and well-being that resonates with your body's intrinsic patterns. This knowledge empowers you to make informed decisions about your health and well-being, attuned to your body's natural rhythms. With this knowledge as a foundation, the next step is to explore the practical aspects of tracking the menstrual cycle, which will empower you to apply this understanding to your own life.

Tracking Your Cycle: Methods and Tools

The next step after learning about hormonal changes and their functions is tracking your cycle. This process is not only fundamental to the process of cycle synchronization but also vital for gaining insights into your health and well-being.

To start tracking your cycle, you'll need to become familiar with the different phases and the length of your menstrual cycle, which can vary from the typical 28-day cycle. The first day of bleeding is considered day one of your cycle, and tracking continues to the day before your next period begins. Here are some ways you can track your cycle:

- **Calendar:** One of the simplest methods to track your cycle is using a calendar. You can mark the first day of your period and count the days until your next period begins. This will give you the length of your cycle. Additionally, you can note any symptoms you experience, such as cramps, mood swings, or changes in energy levels, which can indicate hormonal fluctuations.
- **Cycle tracking applications:** If you prefer to use technology, there are numerous apps available that can assist with cycle tracking. These apps often provide additional features such as reminders, symptom tracking, and predictions for fertile windows, which can be particularly useful for those trying to conceive or avoid pregnancy.
- **Basal body temperature:** Another tool for tracking your cycle is basal body temperature (BBT) charting. Your BBT is your body's temperature at rest and can be an indicator of ovulation. After ovulation, progesterone causes a slight increase in BBT. By tracking this temperature daily, you can see patterns and identify the ovulatory phase of your cycle.
- **Cervical mucus observation:** The consistency and amount of cervical mucus changes throughout your cycle due to

hormonal variations. By tracking these changes, you can learn to recognize the fertile phase of your cycle.
- **Hormone tests**: Hormone testing kits are available for those seeking a more in-depth analysis. These kits can measure hormone levels in your urine to provide information about your cycle, such as when you enter your fertile window or confirm if ovulation has occurred.

It's important to note that while these methods can be very effective, they require consistency and attention to detail. Becoming comfortable with tracking and noticing patterns may take a few cycles. However, the insights gained from this practice can be incredibly empowering. By understanding your body's natural rhythms, you can make more informed decisions about your health, plan your schedule to align with your cycle phases and optimize your well-being.

As you become more attuned to your body's signals and the nuances of your menstrual cycle, you'll be better prepared to delve into the science of cycle alignment and harmonize your lifestyle with the ebbs and flows of your hormonal landscape. This knowledge is a foundation for the next steps in your journey toward a more synchronized and harmonious existence with your body.

Common Myths and Misconceptions

In the journey to understand and harness the power of our menstrual cycles, it is crucial to dismantle the barriers of misinformation that often cloud our perception of them. These can range from benign misunderstandings to deeply ingrained stereotypes.

One common myth is that the menstrual cycle only affects a person's mood. While it is true that hormonal fluctuations can influence emotions, the impact of the menstrual cycle is far more comprehensive, affecting physical energy, cognitive function, and even nutritional needs. To view the cycle through the narrow lens of mood swings alone is to overlook the intricate symphony of changes within the body.

Another misconception is that cycle optimization is solely about fertility and contraception. While understanding the menstrual cycle is undoubtedly beneficial for family planning, cycle syncing extends its benefits to various aspects of health and well-being, including stress management, exercise optimization, and dietary adjustments. It is a holistic approach that acknowledges the cyclical nature of the female body.

There is also the mistaken belief that all menstrual cycles are uniform and should conform to a 28-day standard. In reality, cycles can vary significantly in length and characteristics, with a healthy range typically falling between 21 and 35 days. The notion of a "perfect" cycle can lead to unnecessary anxiety and a misalignment between one's unique rhythm and the generalized cycle alignment recommendations.

Furthermore, some may believe that cycle optimization is an unscientific practice rooted more in new-age philosophy than empirical evidence. However, a growing body of research supports the physiological basis for the practice, highlighting the importance of tailoring lifestyle choices to the menstrual cycle's phases to enhance overall health and quality of life.

Lastly, there is the misconception that cycle synchronization is only for those who experience regular cycles. Even individuals with irregular cycles or conditions such as polycystic ovary syndrome (PCOS) can benefit from understanding their body's signals and patterns. Cycle syncing is not a one-size-fits-all solution but a personalized approach that can be adapted to each individual's unique circumstances.

We can pave the way for a more informed and empowered approach to cycle alignment by dispelling these myths and misconceptions. Through this clarity, individuals can truly harness the potential of their menstrual cycles, not only to optimize their daily lives but also to foster a deeper connection with their bodies.

Chapter Summary

- The menstrual cycle is a complex interplay of hormones affecting health and lifestyle, and understanding it can lead to greater self-awareness and well-being.
- The cycle consists of four phases: menstrual, follicular, ovulation, and luteal, each with distinct hormonal changes and bodily responses.
- The menstrual phase involves shedding the uterine lining, with low hormone levels causing symptoms like cramps and mood swings.
- The follicular phase sees rising estrogen levels as ovarian follicles mature, preparing the uterus for potential pregnancy.
- Ovulation is the release of an egg due to a hormone surge, marking the peak of fertility with physical signs like a rise in basal body temperature.
- The luteal phase involves the secretion of progesterone from the corpus luteum to maintain the uterine lining, with the cycle restarting if no fertilization occurs.
- Hormones like FSH, LH, estrogen, and progesterone guide the menstrual cycle, influencing fertility, mood, and overall health.
- Tracking the menstrual cycle using calendars, apps, BBT charting, cervical mucus observation, or hormone testing kits can empower individuals to align their lifestyles with their cycle phases.
- Cycle synchronization involves aligning diet, exercise, and activities with the menstrual cycle's phases for improved health and harmony.
- Common myths about the menstrual cycle include its impact being limited to mood, its relevance only for fertility, the existence of a "perfect" cycle length, and the dismissal of cycle syncing as unscientific.

2
NUTRITION AND YOUR CYCLE

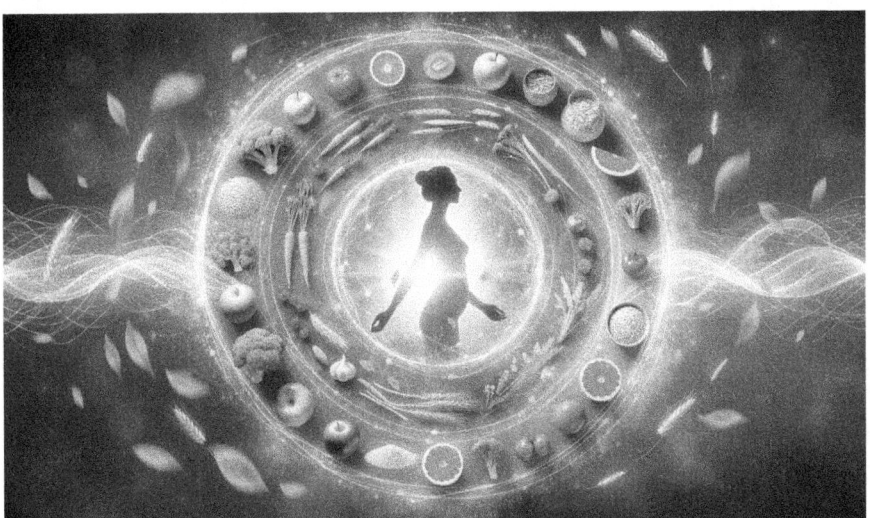

As we begin to explore nutrition and how it relates to your menstrual cycle, it is essential to understand your body's changing nutritional demands during each phase.

Eating for Your Menstrual Phase

As we explored in the last chapter, the menstrual phase marks the beginning of your cycle and is characterized by the shedding of the uterine lining. It can be accompanied by symptoms such as cramps, fatigue, and mood swings and is a period that requires special attention to dietary choices to support your body's needs.

During the menstrual phase, your body is in a state of release and renewal. Iron levels can be particularly impacted due to blood loss, making it crucial to replenish this vital nutrient. Foods rich in iron, like leafy greens, legumes, red meat, poultry, and fish, should be incorporated into your meals. Pair these foods with those high in vitamin C, like citrus fruits, bell peppers, and berries, to enhance iron absorption. This synergistic effect maximizes iron uptake and supports your immune system.

In addition to iron, your body will benefit from foods high in omega-3 fatty acids. These essential fats, found in flaxseeds, walnuts, and fatty fish like salmon, can help manage inflammation and alleviate menstrual cramps. They also influence mood regulation, which can be particularly beneficial if you experience emotional shifts during this phase.

Complex carbohydrates are another critical component of eating for your menstrual phase. Whole grains, such as brown rice, quinoa, and oats, provide sustained energy and are rich in B vitamins, essential for energy production and the health of your nervous system. These complex carbs also contribute to a feeling of fullness and can help stabilize blood sugar levels, curbing cravings and mood swings.

Hydration is paramount during the menstrual phase. Drinking plenty of water helps to replace fluids lost during menstruation and can aid in reducing bloating. Herbal teas, such as ginger or peppermint, can offer additional comfort, easing digestive discomfort and soothing cramps.

Lastly, listening to your body's signals during this time is important. If you experience cravings, it's not uncommon to seek out comfort in the form of food. While it's perfectly acceptable to indulge mindfully, aim to maintain a balance by choosing nutrient-dense snacks like dark chocolate, which is high in magnesium. This mineral can relax muscles and ease cramping.

Focusing on these nutritional strategies during the menstrual phase supports your body's natural processes and sets a strong foundation for the remainder of your cycle. With thoughtful food choices, you can navigate this phase with greater ease and comfort, readying yourself for the transition into the next phase of your cycle, where different nutritional considerations will come into play.

Eating for Your Follicular Phase

As we transition from the menstrual phase into the follicular phase of your cycle, your body embarks on a new beginning. This phase, typically lasting from about day 7 to day 14 of your cycle, is characterized by the body's preparation for potential pregnancy. It's a time when the follicles in the ovaries mature and estrogen levels rise. With this physiological shift, your nutritional needs also evolve.

The follicular phase is an opportune moment to support your body with foods that enhance estrogen production and follicle growth. A diet rich in phytoestrogens can be particularly beneficial during this time. Phytoestrogens are plant-derived compounds that can mimic the effects of estrogen in the body, and they can be found in foods such as flaxseeds, soybeans, and legumes. Incorporating these into your meals can help balance your hormones naturally.

As estrogen levels increase, so does your body's capacity to build muscle. The follicular phase is excellent for focusing on foods rich in high-quality proteins. Think lean meats, fish, eggs, and plant-based sources like quinoa and lentils. These will support muscle growth and repair and provide sustained energy levels.

Your energy levels are likely to be higher during the follicular phase, and your metabolism may also start to speed up. Complex carbohydrates are your allies to match this increased energy demand. They provide a steady release of energy, perfect for keeping you fueled throughout the day. Foods such as sweet potatoes, oats, and whole grains are excellent choices.

Moreover, the follicular phase is when your body is more insulin-sensitive, meaning it's better at utilizing carbohydrates for energy rather than storing them as fat. This makes it a strategic time to include moderate portions of healthy carbohydrates.

Antioxidants are also crucial during this phase to help protect the developing follicle from oxidative stress. Brightly colored fruits and vegetables, such as berries, citrus fruits, and leafy greens, are packed with vitamins and antioxidants. They not only support overall health but also contribute to the health of your reproductive system.

In addition to specific food groups, certain vitamins and minerals deserve special attention during the follicular phase. Vitamin E, found in nuts and seeds, can support the growth of the uterine lining. B vitamins, particularly B6 and B9, are essential for hormone balance and can be found in abundance in legumes, whole grains, and dark leafy vegetables.

Lastly, hydration remains a cornerstone of good health. Consuming ample water throughout the day will aid nutrient transport and overall cellular function.

By aligning your nutrition with your follicular phase, you are not only nurturing your body's immediate needs but also setting the stage for a healthier cycle overall. Remember, the key is to listen to your body and provide it with the nutrients required to thrive during each unique phase of your cycle.

Eating for Your Ovulatory Phase

As we transition from the follicular phase into the ovulatory phase of your menstrual cycle, your nutritional needs subtly shift in response to the hormonal changes within your body. The ovulatory phase, typically spanning 3 to 5 days, is characterized by a peak in luteinizing hormone (LH) and follicle-stimulating hormone (FSH), leading to the release of an egg from the ovary. This is a time of heightened fertility and energy, and your diet can play a supportive role in optimizing your well-being during this phase.

During ovulation, estrogen levels are at their highest, sometimes leading to a slight dip in appetite. However, it's essential to maintain a balanced diet to support your body's increased metabolic rate and the potential for conception if that is your goal.

To harness the full potential of your ovulatory phase through nutrition, focus on incorporating foods rich in fiber, antioxidants, and lean protein. These nutrients support the detoxification processes in the liver, which is vital for metabolizing and excreting excess estrogen.

Fiber-rich foods, such as leafy greens, berries, and legumes, are particularly beneficial during this time. They not only aid in digestion but also help regulate blood sugar levels, which can be particularly sensitive due to hormonal fluctuations. Aim for a variety of colorful vegetables and fruits, as they are packed with antioxidants that protect your cells from oxidative stress and support overall reproductive health.

Lean proteins, including fish, chicken, and plant-based options like lentils and chickpeas, provide the amino acids necessary for muscle repair and growth. These proteins are also vital for producing hormones and enzymes that play a role in the ovulatory process.

Additionally, foods rich in B vitamins, such as whole grains and dark leafy vegetables, can be particularly supportive. Vitamin B6, for instance, plays a role in synthesizing neurotransmitters, which can help maintain a positive mood and energy levels.

Omega-3 fatty acids in fatty fish like salmon, flaxseeds, and walnuts are also beneficial during ovulation. They contribute to the health of the cell membranes, which can be beneficial for egg quality and hormonal balance.

Hydration remains a crucial component of your diet during this phase. Adequate water intake is essential for maintaining the health of your cervical mucus, which is vital for fertility. Aim to drink plenty of water throughout the day, and consider incorporating hydrating foods like cucumbers, watermelon, and citrus fruits.

While the ovulatory phase is relatively short, it's a powerful time window in your cycle. You can support your overall health and vitality by choosing foods that align with your body's natural rhythms. Everyone's body is unique, and listening to your needs and responding is essential. If you have specific dietary restrictions or health concerns, consulting with a healthcare provider or a registered dietitian can provide personalized guidance to optimize your nutrition during this phase of your cycle.

As we explore the intricate relationship between your diet and your menstrual cycle, we will next delve into the nutritional strategies that can support you during the luteal phase, when your body prepares for either pregnancy or the onset of menstruation.

Eating for Your Luteal Phase

As we transition from the ovulatory phase of your menstrual cycle, we enter the luteal phase, which usually spans from day 15 to 28 of a typical 28-day cycle. This phase is characterized by the corpus luteum's release of progesterone, which prepares the body for a potential pregnancy. The luteal phase can often bring about various physical and emotional changes, including premenstrual symptoms. During this time, thoughtful nutrition can play a pivotal role in supporting your body's needs.

During the luteal phase, your metabolism may slightly increase, and you might experience heightened hunger. This is a natural response as your body's energy requirements grow. Increase your caloric intake slightly to accommodate this increased requirement, focusing on nutrient-dense foods that provide sustained energy and support hormonal balance.

Complex carbohydrates are particularly beneficial during this phase. Foods such as sweet potatoes, quinoa, brown rice, and oats can help maintain blood sugar levels and provide the necessary B vitamins that aid in the production of serotonin. This neurotransmitter promotes feelings of well-being and can be particularly helpful if you're experiencing mood swings.

Incorporating a variety of high-fiber foods is also crucial. Fiber helps regulate blood sugar and can aid in digestion, which can sometimes become sluggish during the luteal phase. Vegetables like brussels sprouts, broccoli, leafy greens, legumes, and seeds are excellent fiber sources.

Protein intake should remain consistent, focusing on lean proteins such as chicken, turkey, fish, tofu, and legumes. These proteins provide the amino acids necessary for neurotransmitter production, which can help mitigate some of the emotional changes that may occur during this time.

Healthy fats are another cornerstone of eating for your luteal phase. Foods rich in omega-3 fatty acids, such as salmon, flaxseeds, walnuts, and chia seeds, support cellular health and can help reduce inflammation, which may alleviate some premenstrual symptoms.

Magnesium-rich foods like dark chocolate, avocados, nuts, and seeds can be particularly beneficial. Magnesium plays a role in muscle relaxation and may help ease cramps and tension. It's also involved in synthesizing hormones and can support a sense of calm and relaxation.

Hydration remains essential throughout your cycle, but it's especially important to focus on during the luteal phase when some women experience bloating. Drinking plenty of water can reduce water retention and support overall bodily functions.

Lastly, listening to your body's cues during this phase is important. Craving certain foods during your luteal phase may indicate that your body is seeking specific nutrients. Honor these cravings within the context of a balanced diet, and remember that moderation is vital.

By aligning your nutritional choices with the needs of your luteal phase, you can support your body's natural rhythms and potentially ease some of the symptoms associated with this time of the month. In the following section, we will delve into how supplements can further complement cycle alignment efforts, offering additional support to your overall well-being throughout your menstrual cycle.

Supplements and Your Cycle

In aligning your nutrition with your menstrual cycle, understanding the role of supplements is a vital piece of the puzzle. While whole foods should always be the cornerstone of your diet, certain supplements can support your body's unique needs throughout the different phases of your cycle.

As we delve further into the concept of cycle alignment, it's essential to recognize that a delicate interplay of hormones governs each phase of your menstrual cycle. These hormones regulate your cycle and influence your energy levels, mood, and overall well-being. Supplements, when used thoughtfully and under a healthcare professional's guidance, can help optimize this hormonal balance and support your body's natural rhythms.

During the follicular phase, which begins after menstruation, your body is preparing for the possibility of pregnancy. Estrogen levels rise, leading to increased energy and a more robust metabolism. B-complex vitamins can be particularly beneficial to support this phase. They play a crucial role in energy production and can help maintain steady energy levels. Additionally, antioxidants like Vitamin E and selenium can support egg health, which is paramount during this time.

As you transition into the ovulatory phase, the body focuses on releasing an egg for potential fertilization. This is when you might feel at your most energetic and communicative. To support this phase, consider supplements that support hormonal balance and fertility, such as omega-3 fatty acids, which can aid in producing healthy cervical fluid.

Following ovulation, you enter the luteal phase, which we've previously discussed in the context of nutrition. During this time, progesterone becomes the dominant hormone. This shift can sometimes lead to premenstrual symptoms. Magnesium is a supplement that can be particularly helpful during the luteal phase. It plays a role in mood regulation, can alleviate cramps, and supports sleep. Additionally, Vitamin B6 can aid in synthesizing neurotransmitters like serotonin, which may help reduce mood swings and support overall emotional well-being.

Finally, during menstruation, your body is shedding the uterine lining and resetting for the next cycle. Iron is a crucial supplement during this phase, especially for those who experience heavy bleeding, as it helps to replenish the iron lost during menstruation. Vitamin C can aid in iron absorption, so pairing these two can be particularly effective.

It's crucial to remember that supplements are not a one-size-fits-all solution. The doses and combinations should be tailored to your health profile and the specific needs of each phase of your menstrual cycle. Always consult a healthcare provider before starting any new supplement regimen to ensure it's appropriate for your health status and goals.

By integrating supplements into your cycle-syncing practice, you can provide your body with the targeted support to thrive throughout each phase of your menstrual cycle. In conjunction with a balanced diet, this can empower you to harness the natural ebb and flow of your hormones, leading to improved health and vitality.

Chapter Summary

- The menstrual phase requires dietary choices that support the body's needs, including iron-rich foods and vitamin C to enhance iron absorption.
- Omega-3 fatty acids can help manage inflammation and mood swings, while complex carbohydrates provide sustained energy and stabilize blood sugar levels.
- Hydration is crucial, with water and herbal teas aiding in fluid replacement and reducing bloating, and listening to the body's signals for cravings is essential.
- The follicular phase benefits from foods that enhance estrogen production and muscle growth, including phytoestrogens, high-quality proteins, and complex carbohydrates.

- Antioxidants and specific vitamins like E and B support overall health and hormone balance during the follicular phase.
- The ovulatory phase requires a balanced diet with fiber, antioxidants, and lean protein to support metabolic rate and detoxification.
- The luteal phase may increase hunger and metabolism, requiring complex carbohydrates, high-fiber foods, lean proteins, and healthy fats to support the body.
- Supplements can complement cycle-syncing efforts, with specific vitamins and minerals supporting each menstrual cycle phase under healthcare guidance.

3

EXERCISE AND YOUR CYCLE

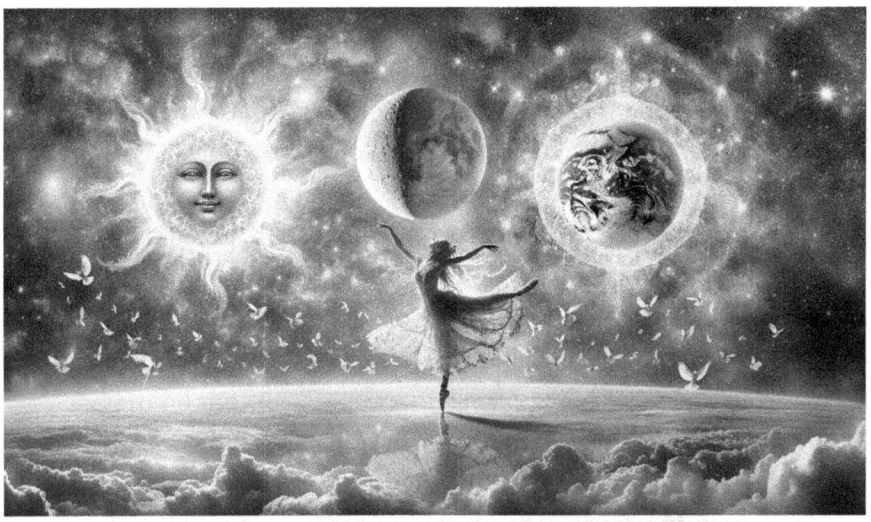

Recognizing the subtle yet informative cues your body provides throughout your menstrual cycle and adapting your workouts to these cues can maximize the benefits you reap from physical exercise. This attunement is the cornerstone of personalizing your fitness routine to harmonize with your cycle.

Adapting Workouts to Your Menstrual Phase

As we delve into the intricacies of cycle synchronization, particularly concerning exercise, it is essential to understand how the menstrual phase of your cycle can influence your workout regimen. During your menstrual phase, your body is shedding the uterine lining, accompanied by symptoms such as cramps, fatigue, and a general feeling of heaviness.

Given these physiological changes, it can help to adapt your exercise routine to accommodate your body's current state. This is not only a matter of comfort, but also one of harnessing the natural rhythm of your energy levels to optimize your fitness outcomes.

During the menstrual phase, your hormone levels—specifically estrogen and progesterone—are at their lowest. This hormonal state can lead to a decrease in energy and strength, making it an opportune time to engage in gentler, restorative workouts. Consider incorporating activities such as:

- **Yoga:** Gentle yoga flows can help to alleviate cramps and soothe your nervous system. Focus on comforting and restorative poses, such as child's pose, cat-cow stretches, and supine twists. These can help ease tension in the lower back and abdominal areas, often where discomfort is most pronounced during menstruation.
- **Walking:** A low-impact activity like walking can maintain your fitness without placing undue stress on your body. It's a form of exercise that can be easily adjusted to your energy levels—whether that means a leisurely stroll or a brisk walk.
- **Swimming:** If you're comfortable with it, swimming can be an excellent way to exercise during your period. The buoyancy of the water supports your body, and the gentle resistance can help maintain muscle tone without the strain of weight-bearing activities.
- **Pilates:** Pilates can help maintain core strength and stability with a low impact on your body. Focusing on breathing and

controlled movements is also beneficial for managing menstrual discomfort.

It's essential to listen to your body during this phase. Light resistance training or a shorter, less intense version of your regular workout might still be appropriate if you feel up to it. However, if your body is signaling the need for rest, honor that. Rest is a critical fitness component, and your body is already working hard during menstruation.

Hydration and proper nutrition are also vital during this phase. Ensure you're drinking plenty of water and eating nutrient-rich foods that can help replenish lost minerals and provide energy.

Remember, the goal of adapting your workouts to your menstrual phase is not to push through discomfort but to align your exercise routine with your body's natural feeling. By doing so, you can maintain your fitness while nurturing your body through the menstrual phase, setting a solid foundation for the more active phases of your cycle.

Adapting Workouts to Your Follicular Phase

As we transition from the menstrual phase into the follicular phase of your cycle, your energy levels begin to rise. This is a time when the body is primed for new beginnings and growth, both metaphorically and physiologically.

During this phase, estrogen levels start to climb, leading to increased energy, better mood, and often a heightened pain threshold. It's an ideal time to capitalize on these physiological changes by adapting your workout routine to match your body's changes. Your follicular is an ideal time to do activities like:

- **Strength training and muscle building:** The rising estrogen levels contribute to a boost in energy and aid in muscle repair and recovery. This makes the follicular phase an ideal time to focus on strength training. You may find that you can lift heavier weights or perform more repetitions than at other

times in your cycle. Incorporate exercises such as squats, deadlifts, and bench presses to build strength and muscle mass. Remember to start with challenging yet manageable weights and progressively increase the load to ensure continuous improvement.
- **Cardiovascular endurance:** Your body's increasing endurance capabilities during the follicular phase make it a great time to engage in more intense cardiovascular activities. Consider adding in running, cycling, or high-intensity interval training (HIIT) sessions. These workouts can help improve your cardiovascular health and take advantage of the natural upswing in your stamina.

As your body is generally less sensitive to pain and discomfort during this phase, it's also beneficial to continue working on flexibility and balance. Incorporate yoga or pilates into your routine to enhance your core strength, flexibility, and balance. These practices support your physical health and can contribute to mental clarity and stress reduction.

With the increase in energy and confidence, the follicular phase is a perfect time to set new fitness goals or try out activities you've been curious about. Whether it's a new fitness class, a challenging hike, or a dance workshop, your body is in an optimal state to embrace and adapt to new physical challenges.

Despite the inclination to push harder during this phase, listening to your body and incorporating adequate rest and recovery is crucial. Ensure you're allowing time for your muscles to repair by taking rest days as needed and engaging in active recovery activities such as light walking or stretching.

To support your increased activity levels, focus on a nutrient-rich diet that includes a balance of carbohydrates for energy, proteins for muscle repair, and healthy fats for hormone production.

By aligning your exercise regimen with the follicular phase of your cycle, you can harness the natural ebb and flow of your energy and hormonal levels. This synchronization optimizes your workouts for better performance and results and fosters a deeper connection with your body's innate wisdom.

Adapting Workouts to Your Ovulatory Phase

As we delve into the ovulatory phase of your menstrual cycle, it's essential to understand how this phase can influence your exercise regimen. The ovulatory phase is when your body is at its peak in terms of energy and physical performance due to a surge in hormones, particularly estrogen and luteinizing hormone. This hormonal shift can significantly impact your workout potential and recovery. You could consider workouts such as:

- **High-intensity and high-impact workouts:** During this phase, your body is primed for high-intensity and high-impact workouts. You may have more stamina, strength, and coordination, making it an excellent time to engage in activities that require power and endurance. This is the phase where you can push your limits and perhaps even set personal records.
- **Strength training:** Strength training during the ovulatory phase can be particularly effective. Due to the peak in estrogen, your muscles are more responsive, and you may experience increased muscle strength and peak power. It's a great time to focus on lifting heavier weights or performing more challenging resistance exercises. However, it's crucial to maintain proper form to prevent injury, as ligaments can be more lax due to hormonal fluctuations.
- **Cardiovascular exercise:** Cardiovascular exercises can also be intensified during this time. Consider incorporating sprint intervals, hill repeats, or high-intensity interval training (HIIT) sessions. These workouts can capitalize on your body's heightened energy levels and improved cardiovascular efficiency.

Group fitness classes or team sports can also be enjoyable and beneficial during ovulation. The social aspect of these activities aligns well with the increased communication skills and confidence often accompanying this phase of your cycle. Engaging with others in a workout setting can provide additional motivation and a sense of camaraderie.

While it's a time to take advantage of your body's peak performance, listening to your body's signals is also essential. Ensure you incorporate adequate warm-up routines to prepare your muscles and joints for intense activity, and don't neglect cool-down periods to aid recovery.

The ovulatory phase presents an opportunity to challenge yourself with higher-intensity workouts, capitalize on your body's increased strength and stamina, and enjoy the social aspects of exercise. By tuning into your body's rhythm and adapting your exercise routine to align with the ovulatory phase, you can optimize your fitness outcomes while honoring the natural rhythm of your cycle.

Adapting Workouts to Your Luteal Phase

As we delve into the luteal phase of your menstrual cycle, it's important to recognize that a shift in energy levels and physical sensations can characterize this period. The luteal phase involves significant hormonal changes that can influence your exercise routine and overall well-being.

During the luteal phase, progesterone levels rise, preparing the body for a potential pregnancy. This increase in progesterone and fluctuating estrogen levels can lead to feelings of bloating, fatigue, and sometimes a decrease in endurance. It's a time when your body is working hard internally, and as such, it may require a different approach to exercise compared to the more energetic ovulatory phase. To adapt your workouts to your luteal phase, consider incorporating the following:

- **Moderate-intensity activities:** These activities support your body's natural rhythms without overtaxing it. Strength training can be particularly beneficial during this time, as it helps maintain muscle mass and bone density. Focus on

moderate weights and higher repetitions rather than striving for personal bests or heavy lifting, which can be more challenging as your energy may not be at its peak.
- **Gentle movement:** Gentle movement practices such as yoga or pilates can be excellent choices. These forms of exercise emphasize core strength, flexibility, and relaxation, which can be soothing if you're experiencing premenstrual symptoms. The mindful breathing techniques used in these practices can also help manage any stress or mood swings that may arise due to hormonal fluctuations.

If your energy levels are still relatively high, consider continuing with cardiovascular exercises like brisk walking or light jogging. However, avoiding high-intensity interval training (HIIT) or prolonged strenuous activities that could exacerbate fatigue or stress the body unnecessarily during this phase can be helpful.

Above all, listening to your body and respecting its signals is essential. If you're feeling particularly tired or experiencing stronger premenstrual symptoms, it may be a sign to scale back the intensity or duration of your workouts. Restorative activities, such as leisurely walks or stretching sessions, can be just as valuable for your health and well-being during this time.

With its unique demands, the luteal phase offers an opportunity to practice self-care and mindfulness as you engage in physical activity. Remember, the goal is to support your body's needs, not push against them, ensuring you maintain a harmonious balance between movement and rest.

Listening to Your Body: Signs and Signals

The dialogue between your body's signals and your exercise choices is an ongoing process that requires patience, observation, and responsiveness.

Firstly, it is essential to recognize that your body's signs and signals are unique to you. They serve as a personal guide to optimizing your workouts. These signals can manifest in various forms, such as energy levels, muscle fatigue, mood fluctuations, and even sleep quality. By paying close attention to these indicators, you can tailor your exercise intensity and type to align with your body's needs at different phases of your cycle.

During the follicular phase, when estrogen levels rise, you might notice a surge in energy and strength. This is an opportune time to engage in more intense and challenging workouts, such as high-intensity interval training (HIIT) or strength training. Conversely, as you transition into the luteal phase, you may observe an energy shift, prompting you to consider more moderate or therapeutic activities, such as yoga or light cardio.

It is also vital to heed the signals of premenstrual syndrome (PMS), which can include bloating, headaches, and mood swings. These symptoms can affect your motivation and comfort during exercise. Adjusting your routine to include gentle movement and stretching can alleviate some of these discomforts and help maintain consistency in your fitness journey.

Moreover, during your menstrual phase, you might experience cramps and lower back pain, which are clear indicators that your body is asking for rest and recovery. This is a time to honor your body's request for gentler practices, perhaps focusing on activities like walking or Pilates, which can help maintain circulation without overexertion.

Listening to your body also means recognizing when you are capable of more than you might initially think. There may be days within each phase of your cycle when you feel powerful and resilient. Embrace these moments by challenging yourself while remaining within the boundaries of what feels right for your body.

In addition to physical signs, emotional and mental signals are equally important. Your mental state can significantly influence your physical performance and vice versa. Acknowledging and respecting your emotional well-being can guide you in choosing an exercise that benefits your body and uplifts your spirit.

Keeping a journal can be incredibly beneficial to facilitate this process of listening. Documenting your physical sensations, emotional state, and energy levels in relation to your cycle can help you discern patterns and make more informed decisions about your exercise regimen.

Remember that cycle alignment is not a one-size-fits-all approach. It is a personalized method that evolves with you as you learn to interpret and honor the signs and signals your body communicates. By doing so, you not only enhance your physical fitness but also foster a deeper connection with your body, leading to a more balanced and fulfilling lifestyle.

Chapter Summary

- The menstrual phase affects exercise routines; engaging in gentler workouts can be helpful due to low energy and strength from decreased estrogen and progesterone levels.
- Recommended activities during menstruation include gentle yoga, walking, swimming, and Pilates to accommodate the body's need for rest and recovery.
- During the follicular phase, rising estrogen levels lead to increased energy and pain tolerance, making it ideal for strength training and intense cardiovascular workouts
- The follicular phase is also an excellent time to focus on flexibility and balance, set new fitness goals, and try new activities while ensuring proper rest and nutrition.
- With a surge in hormones, the ovulatory phase is optimal for high-intensity and high-impact workouts, focusing on strength training and cardiovascular exercises.
- Group fitness and team sports can be enjoyable during the ovulatory phase, but it's essential to warm up properly and stay hydrated and nourished.
- In the luteal phase, rising progesterone may cause bloating and fatigue, so moderate-intensity activities like strength

training with moderate weights and gentle yoga or Pilates are recommended.
- Listening to your body's unique signals throughout the cycle is crucial for tailoring workouts, with attention to physical, emotional, and mental cues, and journaling can aid in recognizing patterns.

4

CYCLE ALIGNMENT IN YOUR PERSONAL LIFE

Social Engagements and Your Cycle

Understanding the nuances of your menstrual cycle can be a transformative tool for organizing your social life. The concept of cycle alignment is not just limited to dietary adjustments or exercise routines; it extends into the realm of your social engagements, providing a useful framework for when to schedule activities, how to interact with others, and even how to manage your energy levels during various phases of your cycle.

During the follicular phase, which begins right after menstruation, your body is gearing up for potential conception. Estrogen levels are rising, leading to increased energy, brain function, and a more outgoing disposition. This is an excellent time to plan social outings, networking events, or any activity that requires active engagement and high energy. You may be more open to new experiences and meeting new people during this phase.

As you transition into the ovulatory phase, communication skills typically peak due to the high estrogen and luteinizing hormone levels. This is an excellent time to have meaningful conversations, attend social gatherings, or give presentations. Your charisma and articulacy are at their highest, making this the optimal time for activities that require verbal communication and social finesse.

The luteal phase, which follows ovulation, can be a bit more complex. In the early part of this phase, you may still enjoy the benefits of high energy and sociability. However, as you move closer to menstruation, your body begins to prepare for a potential pregnancy or to shed the uterine lining. Energy levels may wane, and you might feel more inclined to turn inward. This is a period when you might prefer smaller, more intimate gatherings or quiet evenings at home. It's also a time to be mindful of your emotional state, as some may experience heightened sensitivity or mood swings due to fluctuating hormone levels.

Finally, during menstruation, your body is in a state of release and renewal. Energy is typically at its lowest, and this is a time for rest and reflection. Limiting social engagements during this phase and giving yourself permission to say no to invitations is perfectly acceptable. Focus on self-care and activities that allow for rejuvenation. It's a time to listen to your body and honor its need for rest.

By aligning your social calendar with your menstrual cycle, you can harness the natural levels of your energy and emotions. This doesn't mean you must rigidly follow these guidelines; life is unpredictable, and flexibility is key. However, awareness of your cycle can empower you to make choices that enhance your mental well-being and social satisfaction. It's about working with your body, rather than against it, to create a harmonious balance in your personal life.

Sex and Intimacy: Syncing with Your Partner

Understanding and harmonizing with our menstrual cycle can be profoundly transformative in the realm of personal relationships, particularly with our intimate partners. Cycle synchronization applies not only to our social lives and self-care routines but also extends into the intimate sphere of sex and relationships. By aligning our awareness of the hormonal fluctuations throughout the menstrual cycle with our sexual and emotional needs, we can foster a deeper connection with our partners and enhance our overall well-being.

During the menstrual phase, when energy levels are lower and the body is going through a renewal process, it is natural for some to experience decreased libido. This is a time for open communication with your partner about your needs for comfort and support. Intimacy during this phase doesn't have to be solely about sexual activity; it can also be about cultivating closeness through gentle touch, warm embraces, or simply being in each other's presence.

As you transition into the follicular phase, your energy begins to rise, and so does your potential for sexual desire. This is an excellent time to engage in more active dates and explore new experiences together, both inside and outside the bedroom. The increase in estrogen makes this a prime time for emotional openness and trying new things, which can include experimenting with different forms of sexual expression.

The ovulatory phase often brings with it a peak in libido due to the surge in hormones like estrogen and testosterone. Communication can become more effortless, making you feel more connected to your partner. It's a time when many feel their most confident and expressive, making it an opportune moment to express desires and enjoy a heightened sense of intimacy.

Finally, during the luteal phase, as the body prepares for the possibility of pregnancy or the onset of the menstrual phase, some may experience premenstrual syndrome (PMS), which can affect mood and desire. During this time, remember to be patient with yourself and communicate any emotional or physical needs to your partner. This phase can be a time for deeper emotional bonding and nurturing intimacy in ways that are less physically demanding but equally fulfilling.

Sharing your cycle with your partner and discussing how it impacts your feelings and desires can create a shared understanding and a more empathetic approach to intimacy. It's not about adhering strictly to a schedule but about using the knowledge of your cycle to enhance communication and connection with your partner.

Remember, every individual's experience with their cycle is unique, and it's about finding what works best for you and your partner and using the understanding of your cycle as a tool to support each other's needs and deepen your bond.

Self-Care and Pampering Throughout the Cycle

In the journey of embracing cycle alignment, self-care and pampering are rewarding activities that can enhance your quality of life and fortify your connection with your body's natural rhythms. This practice of aligning self-care routines with the different phases of your menstrual cycle can be both a source of comfort and a tool for empowerment.

During the menstrual phase, when energy levels typically wane and the body calls for rest, it is essential to honor this inward pull. This is a time for gentle self-care. Consider warm baths infused with calming essential oils such as lavender or chamomile, which can soothe the body and the mind. Engage in restorative yoga or light stretching that honors your body's need for rest rather than pushing through high-intensity activities. Embrace the slower pace by curling up with a good book or practicing meditation and deep breathing exercises to center your thoughts and emotions.

As you transition into the follicular phase, your energy begins to rise. Capitalize on this increase by integrating more invigorating self-care practices. This might be the perfect time to try out a new fitness class or engage in creative activities that align with this phase's heightened mental clarity and enthusiasm. Pampering yourself could include a revitalizing facial or a massage that stimulates circulation, complementing the body's natural uptick in energy.

The ovulatory phase allows one to focus on self-care practices that foster connection and expression. This is when you might feel most social and communicative, so consider scheduling appointments for haircuts or beauty treatments that make you feel most confident and radiant. It's also an opportune moment to engage in activities that involve others, like group dance classes or social gatherings, which can be a form of self-care in their own right.

Finally, during the luteal phase, as the body prepares for the possibility of pregnancy or the onset of menstruation, you might experience more physical and emotional sensitivity. This is a time to be particularly gentle with yourself. Opt for self-care that grounds and stabilizes, such as a warm stone massage, acupuncture, or simply ensuring you have ample time for rest. Nutrition also plays a crucial role in self-care during this phase; focus on nourishing foods that support your body's needs, such as magnesium-rich leafy greens and complex carbohydrates, to help manage energy levels and mood.

Incorporating these tailored self-care practices into your routine not only honors your body's natural cycle but also reinforces a nurturing relationship with yourself. By listening to and respecting your body's signals, you create a foundation of well-being that supports you in all facets of life. Remember, the essence of cycle alignment in self-care is about making space for your needs and embracing your body's natural fluctuations with grace and kindness.

Emotional Well-being and Hormonal Fluctuations

The interplay between emotional well-being and hormonal fluctuations is highly relevant to understanding and fully reaping the benefits of cycle alignment. Our hormones are not just biological substances; they are the conductors of the orchestra that is our body, influencing our emotions, energy levels, and overall sense of well-being. We can harness our innate rhythms to foster emotional balance and resilience by tuning into these hormonal cues across our cycle.

During the menstrual phase, when both estrogen and progesterone are at their lowest, you might experience a sense of withdrawal or introspection. It's a time when some may feel more sensitive or prone to introspection. This is a natural period for reflection, and it's beneficial to allow yourself the space to process your emotions, perhaps by journaling or engaging in gentle, meditative activities.

As you transition into the follicular phase, estrogen rises, leading to an increase in energy and a more upbeat mood. The boost in confidence and creativity can be channeled into personal growth and exploration. This is an opportune time to tackle new projects and engage in social activities. Embrace this phase by setting intentions and goals, knowing your body is primed to support you in these endeavors.

The ovulatory phase is often marked by a peak in estrogen and the presence of luteinizing hormone, which can result in feeling more communicative and connected with others. It's a period where you might be more emotionally open and articulate. Leveraging this time for meaningful conversations and fostering relationships can be incredibly fruitful.

Finally, the luteal phase, which leads to menstruation, is characterized by higher progesterone levels. This shift can bring about a more reflective state and a tendency towards nesting and nurturing for some. It's not uncommon to experience premenstrual syndrome (PMS), where emotions can feel more intense or volatile. Recognizing these patterns allows you to plan for self-care strategies to mitigate stress and provide comfort.

By syncing your life with your cycle, you can anticipate and use these emotional shifts to your advantage. It's about creating a personal toolkit that aligns with your hormonal landscape—knowing when to push forward with vigor and when to pull back and replenish. This approach does not suggest that you are at the mercy of your hormones but rather that you can work with them to cultivate a harmonious balance in your emotional life.

Remember, every individual's experience with their cycle is unique. It's essential to observe your patterns and responses. Keeping a cycle diary can be invaluable in this process, helping you identify trends and tailor your approach to cycle syncing to support your emotional well-being best.

By embracing the wisdom of your body's natural rhythms, you can navigate the natural flow of your emotions with grace and self-compassion, leading to a more empowered and harmonious personal life.

Planning Personal Events and Activities by Cycle Phase

Cycle alignment emerges as a transformative approach to harmonize our personal lives with our natural rhythms. We can optimize our energy, productivity, and overall well-being by aligning our personal activities and events with the different phases of our menstrual cycle. This section will guide you through planning your events and activities according to the different phases of your cycle, ensuring that you are working with your body, not against it.

As we explored in earlier chapters, the menstrual phase is usually accompanied by lower energy levels due to the shedding of the uterine lining. It is a time for introspection and rest. This is an excellent opportunity to schedule low-key activities that do not demand high physical exertion, such as gentle yoga, meditation, or simply curling up with a good book. It's also a period for reflection, making it ideal for journaling or planning future goals.

As we transition into the follicular phase, our energy and estrogen levels rise. This is the time to tackle new projects and challenges. It's an excellent phase for brainstorming sessions, starting new hobbies, or planning outings that require more physical activity, such as hiking or cycling. The increase in energy and optimism makes it a favorable time to engage in social activities and network.

The ovulatory phase is often when energy peaks, alongside a surge in communication skills due to the high estrogen and testosterone levels. This is the prime time for important meetings, presentations, or any event where you need to be at your most articulate and charismatic. It's also a great time for social gatherings, parties, or date nights, as you'll likely feel more outgoing and connected.

Finally, the luteal phase, which leads up to menstruation, is characterized by a gradual decline in energy as the body prepares for the potential of pregnancy. This phase can be utilized for completing tasks, following up on projects, and wrapping up loose ends. It's also a period where some may experience premenstrual syndrome (PMS), so it's wise to avoid scheduling highly stressful events or demanding physical challenges. Instead, focus on activities that promote relaxation and self-care, such as a spa day or a creative endeavor that brings you joy.

By syncing your personal life with your cycle, you can create a rhythm that respects your body's natural fluctuations and empowers you to make the most of each phase. With this mindful approach, you can enhance your personal life, ensuring that you are living in a fulfilling and sustainable way.

Chapter Summary

- Cycle alignment can optimize social life by scheduling activities according to the menstrual cycle phases, enhancing energy management and interactions.
- The follicular phase is ideal for high-energy social outings and new experiences due to rising estrogen levels and increased outgoingness.
- The ovulatory phase is best for important conversations and social events, with peak communication skills and charisma due to high estrogen and luteinizing hormone levels.
- Early in the luteal phase can be suitable for socializing, but the latter part is better for intimate gatherings or solitude as energy wanes and mood may fluctuate.
- The menstrual phase is a time for rest and self-care, with reduced social activity and focus on rejuvenation as energy is at its lowest.
- Intimate relationships benefit from cycle syncing, with varying sexual and emotional needs throughout the cycle leading to deeper connections with partners.
- Self-care can be tailored to each cycle phase, with activities ranging from restorative practices during menstruation to energizing and social activities during ovulation.

- Planning your events and activities by cycle phase can enhance productivity and well-being, with each phase offering different opportunities for engagement and rest.
- Hormonal fluctuations influence emotional well-being, and understanding this can help manage emotions and foster resilience throughout the cycle.

5

CYCLE ALIGNMENT IN YOUR PROFESSIONAL LIFE

Productivity and Your Menstrual Cycle

Understanding the intricate relationship between your menstrual cycle and productivity can be a professional game-changer. Cycle synchronization is not just about physical health; it's about harnessing the rhythm of your hormonal landscape to optimize your work life. Let's delve into how the different phases of your menstrual cycle can impact your productivity and how you can leverage this knowledge to your advantage.

As we explored in previous chapters, each phase of the cycle comes with its own set of hormonal fluctuations that can influence your energy levels, cognitive functions, and overall work performance.

During the menstrual phase, when you typically experience lower energy levels, you may prefer to engage in less demanding tasks and introspection. This could be an opportune moment to reflect on your work goals, evaluate past performances, and plan ahead. While it might not be the time for aggressive brainstorming sessions or high-stakes negotiations, it's ideal for setting intentions and organizing tasks that require more focus and less physical exertion. Strategic thinking, long-term planning, and evaluating past performance can be done effectively during this time. It's also a period to be gentle with yourself, scheduling fewer meetings and allowing for more flexible deadlines when possible.

As you transition into the follicular phase, a rise in estrogen levels leads to increased energy, improved mood, and sharper cognitive abilities. This is the time to tackle challenging projects, brainstorm innovative ideas, and take on tasks that require more critical thinking and creativity. Your capacity for complex problem-solving is heightened, making it an excellent time for strategic planning and decision-making.

The ovulatory phase is often characterized by a peak in energy and communication skills, thanks to a surge in estrogen and testosterone. This is when you're likely to feel your most confident and articulate. Capitalize on this phase by scheduling important meetings, presentations, and networking events. It's a prime time for collaborative projects and initiatives that require teamwork and leadership.

Finally, during the luteal phase, you might find your focus turning inwards again, with a preference for completing tasks and tying up loose ends. This is a signal to switch gears from the high-energy tasks of the previous weeks to more detail-oriented and organizational activities. It's an excellent time to focus on completing tasks, following up on emails, and setting your agenda for the coming weeks. You may also find this is when you're best at critical analysis and editing work. While you may start to feel a dip in energy as this phase progresses, it's an opportune time to evaluate the outcomes of your efforts and prepare for the quieter, reflective period of the menstrual phase.

By acknowledging and adapting to the natural fluctuations of your menstrual cycle, you can create a work rhythm that not only respects your body's needs but also maximizes your professional potential. This approach to productivity is not about pushing through at all costs; it's about working smarter by aligning your tasks with the innate capabilities of each cycle phase. With this knowledge, you can craft a more harmonious and effective work life, one that empowers you to perform at your best while also honoring your body.

Communication and Collaboration During Different Phases

Understanding the intricacies of your menstrual cycle can be a powerful tool for enhancing communication and collaboration in the workplace. By aligning your professional interactions with the hormonal changes of your cycle, you can optimize your effectiveness and foster better relationships with colleagues.

During the menstrual phase, which marks the beginning of your cycle, you may experience a desire for introspection. This is a time for clear and concise communication. Prioritize essential conversations and allow yourself to listen more. You might find that your capacity for empathy is heightened during this phase, which can be leveraged to strengthen connections with coworkers. However, it can help to set boundaries to ensure you don't become overwhelmed.

As you transition into the follicular phase, your energy begins to rise, and so does your capacity for creative thinking and problem-solving. This is an opportune time to initiate new team projects and brainstorm with your colleagues. Your communication can become more assertive, and you may feel more inclined to lead discussions. Use this time to schedule meetings that require strategic planning and innovative thinking.

The ovulatory phase is often when you're most communicative and charismatic. Your ability to articulate ideas and your openness to collaboration are at their peak. This is the moment to tackle important negotiations, presentations, and networking opportunities. Embrace your persuasive skills and engage in team-building activities. Your natural magnetism during this phase can help inspire and motivate those around you.

Finally, during the luteal phase, as your body prepares for the possibility of pregnancy or the onset of the menstrual phase, you may notice a shift toward a more reflective state. While you may feel less inclined to socialize with others, you can use this time to provide thoughtful feedback and complete tasks that require focus and persistence. Communication may need to be more measured, as you might find yourself more sensitive to feedback or conflict.

By aligning your communication style and collaborative efforts with the natural fluctuations of your cycle, you can work more harmoniously with your biological rhythms and those around you. You can anticipate shifts in your capabilities and preferences, allowing you to approach tasks and interactions with intention.

Navigating workplace dynamics with cycle awareness is a powerful strategy for professional development. By understanding and working with the rhythms of your cycle, you can create a work life that is more productive and more harmonious with your natural rhythms. This holistic approach to professional growth respects your body's needs and career aspirations, leading to a more balanced and fulfilling work experience.

Chapter Summary

- Cycle alignment in the workplace involves aligning work tasks with the menstrual cycle phases to optimize productivity and professional potential.
- The menstrual phase is a time for introspection and planning, suitable for setting professional goals and organizing tasks requiring focus but less physical exertion.
- The follicular phase brings increased energy and cognitive abilities, ideal for tackling challenging projects, brainstorming, and strategic decision-making.
- The ovulatory phase peaks in energy and communication skills, making it the best time for important meetings, presentations, and collaborative projects.
- The luteal phase is excellent for inward focus, completing tasks, and detail-oriented work, with a gradual energy decline as the phase progresses.

- Communication and collaboration in the workplace can be enhanced by understanding and aligning with the hormonal changes of the menstrual cycle.
- Managing energy levels at work according to the menstrual cycle phases can lead to a healthier work-life balance and increased productivity.
- Navigating workplace dynamics with cycle awareness can improve task management, communication, and overall professional development.

6

CYCLE ALIGNMENT AND FERTILITY

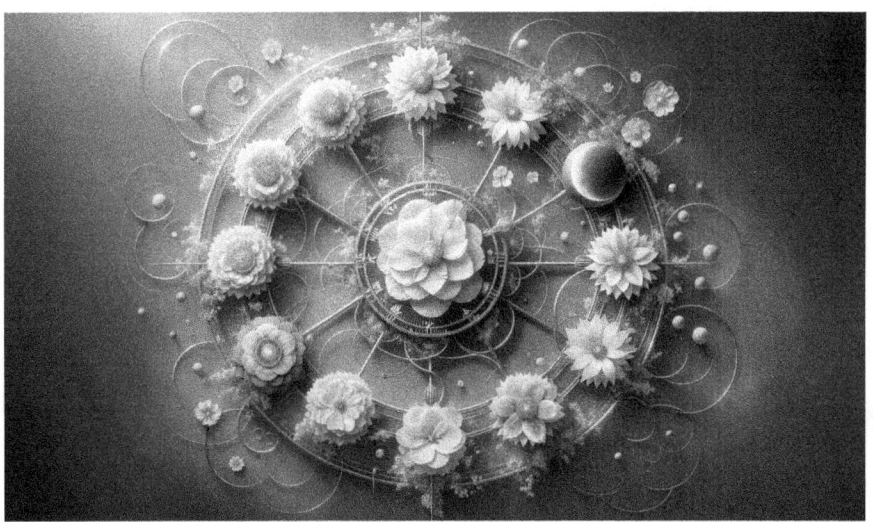

E mbarking on the journey of understanding fertility requires a comprehensive look at the menstrual cycle, a cornerstone of reproductive health. The menstrual cycle is not merely a timekeeper for potential conception; it is a barometer of overall well-being and a window into the intricate workings of the female body.

To grasp the concept of fertility within the cycle, one must first recognize that the menstrual cycle is divided into several phases and the role and contribution of each phase in fertility and contraception.

Ovulation is the pinnacle of fertility within the cycle. It is the moment when the mature egg is released from the ovary and is available for fertilization. The lifespan of the egg is relatively short, typically around 24 hours. Therefore, understanding the timing of ovulation is critical for those aiming to conceive or avoid pregnancy.

Tracking your menstrual cycle and recognizing the signs of each phase is a powerful tool for managing fertility. Body temperature, cervical mucus consistency, and hormonal changes are all indicators that can help pinpoint ovulation. Understanding these signs can help you build cycle alignment habits to optimize your health and achieve fertility goals.

Whether the aim is to enhance fertility or to use natural family planning methods for contraception, knowledge of your cycle is empowering. It allows for a harmonious relationship with the body's natural rhythms, fostering a sense of control and well-being. The next step in this journey is to delve into how cycle alignment can be applied to natural family planning, offering a practical approach to understanding and working with the body's fertility signals.

Natural Family Planning and Cycle Awareness

In understanding one's fertility, cycle awareness is a profound tool for natural family planning. This systematic approach to fertility awareness involves tracking the menstrual cycle to predict ovulation and plan or prevent pregnancy accordingly.

Cycle alignment for natural family planning is based on the principle that a woman is only fertile for a limited number of days during her cycle. By identifying these fertile days, couples can make informed decisions about when to engage in sexual activity, depending on their family planning goals.

The first step in natural family planning with cycle syncing is establishing a baseline understanding of your menstrual cycle. This requires regular observation and documentation over several months. You can record the start and end dates of your periods and any associated symptoms, such as cramping or mood changes, using the methods we discussed in earlier chapters.

Once you've identified your cycle pattern, you can shift your focus to pinpointing ovulation. Numerous physical signs can indicate the approach of ovulation, including changes in cervical mucus, a slight rise in basal body temperature, and even subtle shifts in libido or energy levels. You could also opt to use ovulation predictor kits for more precise identification of your fertile window.

During the fertile window, which typically spans five days leading up to and including the day of ovulation, couples seeking to conceive can increase their chances of pregnancy by having intercourse. Conversely, those who wish to avoid pregnancy can either abstain from sexual activity during this time or use barrier methods of contraception.

It's important to note that cycle syncing for natural family planning requires high commitment and self-awareness. Factors such as stress, illness, and lifestyle changes can all influence the menstrual cycle, potentially affecting the accuracy of fertility predictions. Therefore, paying close attention to your body and any factors that may cause variations in your cycle is beneficial.

This natural family planning method is most effective when cycles are regular and predictable. Women with irregular cycles may find it more challenging to use cycle alignment as a reliable form of natural family planning. They may need to explore additional methods or consult a healthcare professional for guidance.

Empowering yourself with the knowledge of cycle syncing for natural family planning fosters a deeper connection with your body. It provides a sense of control and partnership in the reproductive process. It is a natural, non-invasive approach that, when practiced diligently, can be a powerful ally in the journey of fertility management.

Optimizing Fertility Through Lifestyle Choices

Beyond the biological mechanics, lifestyle choices play a significant role in optimizing fertility. By aligning daily habits with the body's natural rhythms, you can create an environment conducive to conception.

Nutrition is a cornerstone of reproductive health. A diet rich in whole foods provides the necessary vitamins and minerals that support hormonal balance and egg quality. During the follicular phase, when the body is preparing for ovulation, incorporating foods high in antioxidants, such as berries and leafy greens, can aid in protecting the eggs from oxidative stress. As one transitions into the luteal phase, the focus shifts to foods that support progesterone production, like those rich in B vitamins and omega-3 fatty acids, found in whole grains and fatty fish, respectively.

Physical activity, too, should be tailored to the menstrual cycle. During the first half of the cycle, energy levels tend to be higher, making it a suitable time for more vigorous exercises, which can improve blood flow and reduce stress. As the cycle progresses, particularly after ovulation, gentler activities like yoga or walking can help maintain a sense of calm and reduce inflammation without overly taxing the body.

Stress management is another critical element. Chronic stress can disrupt the delicate hormonal interplay necessary for ovulation and implantation. Techniques such as mindfulness meditation, deep-breathing exercises, or engaging in hobbies that bring joy can mitigate stress and promote a more harmonious internal environment.

Sleep quality cannot be underestimated in its importance for fertility. Adequate, restorative sleep helps regulate the hormones that drive the menstrual cycle. Maintaining a consistent sleep schedule and creating a restful sleeping environment can bolster overall health and, by extension, fertility.

Lastly, environmental factors such as exposure to toxins should be minimized. Chemicals in certain plastics, personal care products, and household cleaners can have estrogen-like effects on the body, potentially disrupting hormonal balance. Opting for natural or organic alternatives can reduce this exposure and support the body's natural hormonal rhythms.

You can nurture your fertility by making conscious lifestyle choices that honor your body's cyclical nature. This holistic approach to health supports the physical dimension of conception and fosters a deeper connection with one's own body, empowering individuals on their path to parenthood.

Dealing with Infertility and Cycle Irregularities

Embarking on the journey to conceive can be filled with a spectrum of emotions, from excitement and hope to anxiety and uncertainty. When faced with infertility and cycle irregularities, these feelings can intensify. It's helpful to approach these challenges with a sense of empowerment and a systematic plan to navigate the complexities they present.

Infertility, commonly defined as the inability to conceive after one year of unprotected intercourse for women under 35 or after six months for women over 35, affects many couples worldwide. Cycle irregularities, manifesting as irregular periods, anovulation, or hormonal imbalances, can further complicate the ability to conceive. Understanding and addressing these issues cannot be missed in the journey towards conception.

Aligning lifestyle choices with the different phases of your menstrual cycle can be a valuable tool in managing infertility and cycle irregularities. By becoming attuned to the body's natural rhythms, you can implement targeted strategies that may enhance your fertility.

The first step in dealing with these challenges is to gather comprehensive information. This involves tracking menstrual cycles, noting the length, regularity, and symptoms experienced throughout. Apps and journals can be helpful tools in this process. A thorough understanding of your cycle provides invaluable insights and can help healthcare providers diagnose and treat any underlying issues.

Next, it's essential to seek professional guidance. A fertility specialist can conduct a range of tests to determine the cause of infertility or irregular cycles. These may include blood tests to assess hormone levels, ultrasounds to examine the reproductive organs and other diagnostic procedures. With this information, a tailored treatment plan can be developed, including cycle-syncing techniques, medical interventions, or a combination of both.

For those experiencing cycle irregularities, cycle alignment can be particularly beneficial. One can support hormonal balance and overall reproductive health by focusing on nutrition, exercise, stress management, and sleep patterns in accordance with the menstrual phases. For instance, when estrogen levels rise during the follicular phase, engaging in more intense physical activity and consuming a diet rich in phytoestrogens might be advantageous. Conversely, when progesterone is dominant during the luteal phase, emphasizing stress-reduction techniques and ensuring adequate intake of B vitamins could be more beneficial.

In addition to lifestyle modifications, medical treatments such as hormone therapy or assisted reproductive technologies (ART) may be necessary. These interventions should be considered part of a holistic approach, where cycle alignment plays a supportive role.

It's also important to acknowledge the emotional toll that infertility and cycle irregularities can take. Whether through counseling, support groups, or mindfulness practices, mental health support is a vital component of care. Emotional well-being is intrinsically linked to physical health, and nurturing both is paramount in creating the most supportive environment for conception.

In conclusion, while infertility and cycle irregularities present significant challenges, they are not insurmountable. With a proactive and informed approach, incorporating cycle alignment as a complementary practice and harnessing the expertise of healthcare professionals, individuals, and couples can enhance their fertility potential. By taking control of your health and making informed decisions, the path to parenthood, though sometimes winding, becomes clearer and more navigable.

Preconception Care and Cycle Alignment

Embarking on the journey to parenthood can be a time of great anticipation and, sometimes, anxiety.

Preconception care is a critical phase where potential parents can take proactive steps to enhance their health and well-being, creating the best possible environment for conception. Cycle alignment can be a valuable tool in this preparatory stage.

The menstrual cycle is a barometer of overall health, and its regularity often indicates a balanced hormonal environment. Observing and charting the menstrual cycle allows one to gain insights into their unique hormonal patterns and identify potential issues that could affect fertility. Cycle syncing empowers individuals to work with their bodies, rather than against them, by tailoring their preconception regimen to the natural rhythms of their cycle.

During the follicular phase, which begins after menstruation and leads up to ovulation, estrogen levels rise, and the body prepares for the possibility of pregnancy. This is when energy levels may increase, and the body is more receptive to nutrient-rich foods and moderate to high-intensity exercise. Emphasizing a diet rich in antioxidants, lean proteins, and complex carbohydrates can support egg health and hormonal balance.

As the cycle progresses to ovulation, this is the prime time for conception. Understanding the signs of ovulation, such as changes in cervical mucus and basal body temperature, can help in timing intercourse for the best chances of fertilization. Engaging in gentle stress-reduction techniques like yoga or meditation can also create a more conducive environment for conception.

Following ovulation, the luteal phase begins, marked by the production of progesterone, which prepares the uterine lining for potential implantation. During this phase, the body's basal metabolic rate increases, and additional calories may be needed. Choosing foods high in B vitamins and omega-3 fatty acids can support progesterone levels and reduce inflammation. Lighter exercise, such as walking or pilates, can maintain physical health without overly stressing the body.

In addition to dietary and exercise modifications, preconception care should also address other lifestyle factors that can impact fertility. This includes managing stress levels, as chronic stress can disrupt hormonal balance and menstrual regularity. Adequate sleep, mindfulness practices, and counseling or support groups can be beneficial in maintaining emotional equilibrium.

Environmental toxins are another consideration in preconception care. Exposure to certain chemicals in plastics, personal care products, and household cleaners can interfere with hormonal function. Adopting a more natural, organic lifestyle can reduce these exposures and support overall reproductive health.

Lastly, preconception care is not solely the responsibility of the individual trying to conceive. Partners can also engage in cycle alignment by being supportive and involved in lifestyle changes, understanding the menstrual cycle's phases, and contributing to a stress-free environment conducive to conception.

By integrating cycle syncing into preconception care, individuals and couples can feel empowered in their journey toward fertility. This practical approach allows for a deeper connection with one's body and can pave the way for a healthy pregnancy and beyond. It is a testament to the power of informed, proactive health management and the beauty of working in harmony with the body's natural processes.

Chapter Summary

- The menstrual cycle is a key indicator of reproductive health and overall well-being.
- Ovulation is the peak of fertility in the cycle, with a short egg lifespan, making timing knowledge crucial for conception or contraception.
- Tracking the menstrual cycle's signs, such as body temperature and cervical mucus, aids in cycle syncing to optimize health and fertility goals.

- Cycle syncing for natural family planning involves identifying fertile days to plan or prevent pregnancy, requiring careful cycle observation and documentation.
- Lifestyle choices, including diet and exercise tailored to the menstrual cycle, significantly optimize fertility.
- Infertility and cycle irregularities can be managed by cycle syncing, professional guidance, and possibly medical treatments, with attention to emotional well-being.
- Preconception care with cycle syncing involves aligning diet, exercise, and lifestyle with menstrual phases to prepare the body for pregnancy.
- Partners can support preconception care by understanding the menstrual cycle and contributing to a healthy environment for conception.

7
CYCLE ALIGNMENT FOR HEALTH CONDITIONS

PCOS and Cycle Alignment

Polycystic Ovary Syndrome, commonly known as PCOS, is a condition characterized by hormonal imbalances that can affect a woman's menstrual cycle, fertility, and various aspects of her health. Cycle alignment has emerged as a potential method to help manage the symptoms of PCOS.

In the follicular phase, which starts on the first day of menstruation and lasts until ovulation, women with PCOS may benefit from gentle, low-intensity exercises and focusing on foods that support estrogen production and balance blood sugar levels, including high-fiber foods, lean proteins, and omega-3 fatty acids.

As the cycle progresses into the ovulatory phase, it is often recommended to incorporate foods rich in B vitamins and zinc, which can support ovulation. Moderate-intensity exercises like cycling or swimming can be introduced, as they help boost energy levels and improve mood.

During the luteal phase, which occurs after ovulation and before the start of menstruation, women with PCOS may experience premenstrual syndrome (PMS) symptoms more intensely. To combat this, a diet rich in magnesium, calcium, and fiber can be helpful. These nutrients can be found in leafy greens, nuts, seeds, and whole grains. Stress management techniques, such as deep breathing exercises and mindfulness meditation, can also be beneficial during this time to help manage any mood swings or anxiety.

Finally, in the menstrual phase, focusing on hydration and replenishing iron levels due to blood loss is essential. Iron-rich foods such as lean meats, legumes, and spinach can be incorporated into the diet. Light exercise, such as stretching or restorative yoga, can help alleviate cramps and maintain circulation.

It is crucial to note that while cycle syncing can be a valuable tool for managing PCOS symptoms, it should be approached with individualized care and in consultation with a healthcare provider. Each woman's experience with PCOS is unique, and what works for one may not work for another. Therefore, a personalized approach that considers the individual's specific needs and symptoms is essential.

Moreover, cycle syncing is not a standalone treatment for PCOS. It is most effective when combined with other medical or therapeutic interventions recommended by healthcare professionals. This holistic approach can empower women with PCOS to take charge of their health and well-being, improving their quality of life and alleviating the symptoms associated with this condition.

Endometriosis and Menstrual Health

Endometriosis is a chronic condition that affects an estimated 1 in 10 women during their reproductive years. This condition is characterized by the presence of endometrial-like tissue outside the uterus, which can lead to a myriad of symptoms, including, but not limited to, severe menstrual pain, chronic pelvic pain, and infertility. The complexity of endometriosis and its impact on menstrual health calls for a multifaceted approach to management, one of which may include cycle alignment.

Understanding and adapting to the body's natural rhythms can be particularly empowering for women with endometriosis. It offers a sense of control over a condition that often feels unpredictable and unmanageable.

During the menstrual phase, when cramping and pain can be at their worst for those with endometriosis, a focus on anti-inflammatory foods and gentle movement can provide some relief. Foods rich in omega-3 fatty acids, such as flaxseeds and walnuts, and antioxidant-rich fruits and vegetables can help reduce inflammation. Gentle yoga or walking can maintain circulation and reduce discomfort without exacerbating symptoms.

Ovulation may present a unique set of challenges for those with endometriosis, as this is a time when symptoms can either improve or worsen. Listening to one's body and adjusting activities and diet is essential. Some may find they can maintain increased activity levels, while others may need to back up.

Finally, during the luteal phase, when premenstrual symptoms can mimic or exacerbate endometriosis pain, it's crucial to continue focusing on anti-inflammatory foods and incorporate stress-reduction techniques. Practices such as meditation, deep-breathing exercises, and restorative yoga can help manage stress, which can help regulate hormone levels and potentially reduce symptoms.

It's important to note that cycle syncing is not a cure for endometriosis but rather a complementary approach to help manage symptoms. Each woman's experience with endometriosis is unique, and what works for one may not work for another. Therefore, it's crucial to approach cycle syncing with a spirit of self-exploration and to work closely with healthcare providers to create a personalized plan that considers all aspects of health.

In addition to lifestyle modifications, medical treatments for endometriosis may include hormonal therapies, pain management strategies, and, in some cases, surgery. Cycle alignment can be integrated into a broader treatment plan, offering a holistic approach that empowers women to manage their condition actively.

By aligning lifestyle choices with the menstrual cycle, women with endometriosis can improve their quality of life and better understand their bodies. It's a journey of self-care that acknowledges the intricate connection between our daily habits and menstrual health.

Thyroid Health and Menstrual Regulation

Understanding the intricate dance between thyroid function and menstrual health is a pivotal step in harnessing the power of cycle alignment to manage and potentially improve various health conditions. The thyroid gland, a small butterfly-shaped organ located at the base of your neck, plays a crucial role in regulating metabolism, energy levels, and, importantly for our discussion, the menstrual cycle.

Thyroid hormones, primarily thyroxine (T4) and triiodothyronine (T3) influence the menstrual cycle by interacting with sex hormones. An imbalance in thyroid function can lead to menstrual irregularities such as amenorrhea (absence of menstruation), menorrhagia (heavy menstrual bleeding), or oligomenorrhea (infrequent menstruation). These conditions can be distressing and impact your quality of life, fertility, and overall health.

Cycle alignment can be particularly beneficial for those with thyroid-related menstrual irregularities. By understanding and working with the body's natural rhythms, it is possible to support thyroid health and, as a result, promote more regular menstrual cycles.

The follicular phase is an opportune time to focus on foods that support estrogen metabolism and thyroid function. Including foods rich in iodine, selenium, and zinc, such as seaweed, brazil nuts, and pumpkin seeds, can support thyroid hormone production and conversion.

As the body transitions into the ovulatory phase, the peak in estrogen can be leveraged to support thyroid health through moderate exercise, which can help maintain a healthy weight and reduce stress, both of which are beneficial for thyroid function.

During the luteal phase, some women may experience a slight dip in thyroid hormones. To counteract this, it can help to incorporate stress-reduction techniques such as yoga or meditation, as stress can exacerbate thyroid issues. Additionally, maintaining a consistent intake of complex carbohydrates during this phase can help stabilize blood sugar levels, which is important for both thyroid health and menstrual regularity.

It is important to note that while cycle alignment can be a powerful tool in managing thyroid health and menstrual regulation, it is not a substitute for medical treatment. Those with thyroid conditions such as hypothyroidism or hyperthyroidism should work closely with their healthcare provider to manage their condition, as medication may be necessary.

Incorporating cycle alignment into a holistic approach that includes medical treatment, when necessary, can empower women to take charge of their health. By understanding the interplay between the thyroid and menstrual cycle, women can make informed choices that support their well-being throughout the entire menstrual cycle.

As we explore the potential of cycle alignment for various health conditions, it becomes clear that awareness and personalization are key. Just as each woman's cycle is unique, so is how her body will respond to different phases and the strategies she can employ to support her health. With this knowledge, we can move forward to address premenstrual syndrome (PMS) and premenstrual dysphoric disorder (PMDD). These conditions also benefit from a deeper understanding of the menstrual cycle and its connection to overall health.

Managing PMS and PMDD with Cycle Awareness

Premenstrual Syndrome (PMS) and Premenstrual Dysphoric Disorder (PMDD) are two health conditions that can significantly impact a woman's quality of life. While PMS is more common and its symptoms are typically milder, PMDD is a severe form of PMS that can be debilitating. Both conditions manifest in the luteal phase of the menstrual cycle, which is the period after ovulation and before the start of menstruation. Cycle alignment can be a powerful tool in managing the symptoms of PMS and PMDD.

Understanding the hormonal fluctuations that characterize the menstrual cycle is the first step in cycle syncing for PMS and PMDD. During the luteal phase, estrogen levels decline while progesterone levels rise and fall if pregnancy does not occur. It is these hormonal shifts that are thought to trigger the symptoms of PMS and PMDD. Symptoms can range from mood swings, bloating, and breast tenderness to more severe psychological symptoms such as anxiety and depression in the case of PMDD.

By becoming cycle-aware, women can anticipate the onset of these symptoms and implement strategies to mitigate them. For instance, dietary adjustments can play a significant role in symptom management. Focusing on foods rich in B vitamins, calcium, magnesium, and omega-3 fatty acids during the luteal phase can help alleviate mood swings and physical discomfort. Additionally, reducing the intake of caffeine, alcohol, and high-sodium foods may decrease bloating and fluid retention.

Stress management techniques are also crucial during this phase. Practices such as mindfulness meditation, deep-breathing exercises, and journaling can help manage the emotional symptoms associated with PMS and PMDD. Sleep hygiene is equally important; adequate rest can help regulate mood and improve overall well-being.

For those with PMDD, where symptoms are more severe and disruptive, it may be necessary to work with a healthcare provider to develop a comprehensive treatment plan. This plan could include cycle alignment strategies and other interventions such as cognitive-behavioral therapy or medication.

In conclusion, cycle synchronization offers a proactive approach to managing the symptoms of PMS and PMDD. By understanding and working with the body's natural rhythms, women can empower themselves to take control of their well-being. It is a systematic and personalized strategy that can be adjusted as needed, providing a sense of agency over one's health. As we move forward, we will explore how stress, which can be both a trigger and an amplifier of menstrual symptoms, interacts with the menstrual cycle and what strategies you can use to mitigate its effects.

The Impact of Stress on Your Menstrual Cycle

To understand how various factors influence menstrual health, it is crucial to address the role of stress, a pervasive element in modern life that can significantly affect your menstrual cycle. Stress, whether acute or chronic, can disrupt the delicate hormonal balance that regulates the menstrual cycle, leading to a range of symptoms and conditions that may compromise overall well-being.

The menstrual cycle is orchestrated by a symphony of hormones, primarily estrogen and progesterone, sensitive to stress-induced changes. When you experience stress, your body produces higher cortisol levels, a hormone released by the adrenal glands. Cortisol is often called the "stress hormone" because it helps your body manage and adapt to stress. However, when cortisol levels are consistently elevated, it can lead to a hormonal imbalance, affecting the production and regulation of reproductive hormones.

This hormonal disruption can manifest in various ways. For some, it may cause irregularities in the menstrual cycle, such as missed periods or unpredictable menstrual flow. For others, stress can exacerbate premenstrual symptoms, making the days leading up to menstruation particularly challenging. In more severe cases, chronic stress can contribute to the development of conditions such as amenorrhea and the absence of menstruation or can worsen the symptoms of polycystic ovary syndrome (PCOS).

Understanding the impact of stress on your menstrual cycle is the first step towards mitigating its effects. By recognizing the times when you may be more vulnerable to stress, you can implement strategies to bolster resilience and maintain hormonal balance.

During the follicular phase, when estrogen levels are rising, you may be more capable of handling stress due to the uplifting effects of this hormone. Conversely, when progesterone is dominant during the luteal phase, you may feel more inclined towards introspection and rest. Honoring these natural rhythms by adjusting your workload and stress management techniques can help maintain hormonal equilibrium.

Practical stress-reduction strategies include mindfulness meditation, deep-breathing exercises, regular physical activity, and ensuring adequate sleep. Nutrition is also pivotal in managing stress and supporting the menstrual cycle. A balanced diet rich in whole foods, emphasizing magnesium, vitamin B6, and omega-3 fatty acids, can provide the necessary nutrients to support your body's stress response and hormonal health.

By acknowledging the profound impact of stress on the menstrual cycle and adopting cycle alignment as a proactive approach to wellness, you can create a supportive environment for your body to thrive. This helps manage stress-related menstrual irregularities and empowers you to harness your body's innate wisdom, leading to improved health outcomes and a greater sense of harmony with your natural cycles.

Chapter Summary

- The symptoms of health conditions such as PCOS and endometriosis can be managed with cycle alignment, tailoring diet and exercise to menstrual phases, starting with estrogen-supportive foods and gentle exercise in the follicular phase.
- Thyroid health and menstrual regulation can benefit from cycle alignment, focusing on supporting thyroid function through diet and stress management across different menstrual phases.
- Managing symptoms of PMS and PMDD involves cycle awareness, dietary adjustments, tailored exercise, stress management, and possibly medical interventions for severe cases.
- Stress, whether acute or chronic, can disrupt the delicate hormonal balance that regulates your menstrual cycle and lead to a range of symptoms and conditions that may compromise your well-being.

- Acknowledging the profound impact of stress on the menstrual cycle and adopting cycle alignment as a proactive approach to wellness can help you create a supportive environment for your body to thrive.

8

HOLISTIC APPROACHES TO CYCLE ALIGNMENT

Integrating Mindfulness and Meditation

In the journey toward harmonizing with our body's natural rhythms, mindfulness, and meditation emerge as powerful tools for cycle syncing. These practices offer a pathway to deeper self-awareness and can significantly enhance our connection to the ebbs and flows of our menstrual cycle.

At its core, mindfulness is the practice of being fully present and engaged in the moment, aware of our thoughts and feelings without distraction or judgment. When applied to cycle syncing, mindfulness encourages us to tune into our body's signals and recognize the subtle shifts that occur throughout the different phases of our menstrual cycle. By observing these changes with a non-judgmental attitude, we can better understand our patterns and respond to our body's needs with compassion and care.

Meditation, a complementary practice to mindfulness, involves sitting quietly and focusing the mind, often on a particular object, thought, or activity, to achieve mental clarity and emotional calmness. During the menstrual cycle, meditation can be tailored to address the specific needs of each phase. For instance, during the menstrual phase, when energy may be lower, a guided visualization focused on rest and renewal can be particularly soothing. Conversely, when energy levels are typically higher during the ovulatory phase, a meditation centered on empowerment and creativity can help harness this vibrant energy.

Integrating mindfulness and meditation into cycle syncing not only aids in managing physical symptoms but also supports emotional well-being. It can help alleviate stress, which disrupts hormonal balance and promotes a sense of peace and grounding. This, in turn, can lead to more balanced cycles and a more profound sense of harmony with one's body.

To begin incorporating these practices, you could start with a simple daily mindfulness exercise, such as paying attention to your breathing or conducting a body scan to notice any areas of tension or ease. This can be done at any time of day and adjusted to fit into your schedule. Meditation can also be introduced gradually, with five to ten-minute sessions focusing on themes relevant to the current menstrual phase.

As we delve deeper into the holistic approaches to cycle syncing, it becomes evident that nurturing our menstrual health extends beyond the realm of the mind. The natural world offers a bounty of herbal remedies that have been used for centuries to support women's health. In the following discussion, we will explore how these herbal allies can be integrated into a holistic strategy for menstrual wellness, complementing the mindful practices of meditation and cycle awareness.

Herbal Remedies and Menstrual Health

Many individuals are turning toward the wisdom of herbal remedies to achieve a harmonious relationship with one's menstrual cycle. This ancient practice, deeply rooted in the knowledge of natural healers and traditional medicine, offers many options for those seeking to support their menstrual health through cycle syncing.

Herbs have been used for centuries to address various health issues, including those related to the menstrual cycle. Their application in cycle syncing is based on the understanding that different menstrual cycle phases may benefit from specific herbal support to optimize overall well-being.

During the follicular phase, the body is preparing for the possibility of ovulation and pregnancy. Herbs that support estrogen production and follicle growth can be particularly beneficial during this time. For example, Vitex agnus-castus, commonly known as chasteberry, is often recommended to help regulate hormonal imbalances and promote a healthy menstrual cycle.

As the cycle progresses into the ovulatory phase, the focus shifts to herbs that support the luteinizing hormone surge and the release of the egg. Herbs like Shatavari (Asparagus racemosus) and Evening Primrose Oil are known for their supportive role in enhancing fertility and maintaining hormonal balance.

The luteal phase, which follows ovulation, is when the body prepares for the potential of pregnancy or transitions into the menstrual phase. During this phase, herbs that support progesterone levels are key. For instance, Cimicifuga racemosa, also known as black cohosh, has been traditionally used to ease premenstrual symptoms and support the cycle's luteal phase.

Finally, during menstruation, the body benefits from herbs that can help alleviate cramps, regulate blood flow, and soothe the system. Ginger (Zingiber officinale) and Cramp Bark (Viburnum opulus) are two such herbs that have been revered for their effectiveness in reducing menstrual discomfort and supporting a healthy menstrual flow.

It is important to approach herbal remedies with an understanding of their potency and potential interactions with other medications. Consulting with a healthcare provider, particularly one specializing in herbal medicine or naturopathy, is essential before integrating these remedies into one's cycle alignment routine. This ensures personalized advice that considers individual health histories and current conditions.

Moreover, the quality of herbal supplements is paramount. Sourcing herbs from reputable suppliers and opting for organic, non-GMO options whenever possible can significantly enhance their therapeutic benefits.

Attention to preparation and dosage is also crucial, as the efficacy of herbal remedies can vary greatly depending on these factors.

Incorporating herbal remedies into cycle alignment is not merely about addressing symptoms; it is about nurturing the body's natural rhythms and fostering a deeper connection with one's cyclical nature. By mindfully selecting and utilizing herbs that resonate with the different phases of the menstrual cycle, individuals can empower themselves to support their menstrual health in a holistic and nurturing manner.

As we explore holistic approaches to cycle alignment, the integration of various modalities becomes apparent. The next step in this journey delves into the ancient practice of Acupuncture and Traditional Chinese Medicine, which offers another layer of depth to understanding and supporting menstrual health.

Acupuncture and Traditional Chinese Medicine

In holistic health, acupuncture and Traditional Chinese Medicine (TCM) are time-honored practices with a rich tapestry of methods for addressing various health concerns, including menstrual health and cycle alignment. These ancient modalities offer a unique perspective on the body's energetic balance and provide tools for aligning one's cycle with the body's natural rhythms.

Acupuncture, a key component of TCM, involves the insertion of fine needles into specific points on the body to stimulate the flow of Qi or vital energy. According to TCM theory, the menstrual cycle is governed by the ebb and flow of this energy and the balance of the Yin and Yang forces within the body. By targeting acupuncture points linked to the reproductive organs, practitioners aim to harmonize these forces and promote a regular, pain-free menstrual cycle.

For those seeking to sync their cycles with their lifestyles, acupuncture can be particularly beneficial during different menstrual cycle phases. During the menstrual phase, for instance, acupuncture may focus on points that help to alleviate cramps and regulate blood flow. In the follicular phase, treatments aim to enhance energy levels and support the growth of the uterine lining. The ovulatory phase may emphasize points that encourage ovulation and fertility. In contrast, the luteal phase treatments could target points to alleviate symptoms of premenstrual syndrome (PMS) and support the potential early stages of pregnancy.

Beyond acupuncture, TCM also encompasses a holistic view of diet and lifestyle, advocating for a diet that supports menstrual health. Foods are chosen based on their energetic properties and ability to nourish the blood, support the Qi, and maintain the balance of Yin and Yang. For example, during the menstrual phase, it is suggested to consume warm, iron-rich foods to replenish lost blood and energy. In contrast, foods that support liver and kidney function, which are believed to be closely tied to reproductive health, are emphasized during the ovulatory phase.

Additionally, TCM practitioners may recommend specific exercises and practices that align with the energetic qualities of each menstrual phase. Gentle movements and breathing exercises can help maintain Qi's smooth flow throughout the body, which is essential for a balanced cycle.

It is important to note that while acupuncture and TCM offer a holistic approach to cycle syncing, they should be pursued with the guidance of a qualified practitioner. This ensures the treatments are tailored to the individual's unique constitution and health needs. Moreover, it is advisable to integrate these practices with conventional medical advice, particularly for those with underlying health conditions or those who are taking medications.

In summary, acupuncture and Traditional Chinese Medicine provide a comprehensive framework for understanding and nurturing menstrual health through cycle alignment. By considering the body's energetic landscape and employing targeted interventions, these practices aim to foster a harmonious menstrual cycle that resonates with the body's innate wisdom and the individual's lifestyle.

Yoga and Cycle Syncing

In the pursuit of aligning one's lifestyle with the intricacies of the menstrual cycle, yoga emerges as a potent ally. This ancient practice, rooted in the harmonization of body and mind, offers a dynamic approach to cycle syncing that can be tailored to the shifting phases of the menstrual cycle. By understanding the unique needs of each phase, individuals can employ specific yoga practices to support hormonal balance and overall well-being.

During the menstrual phase, when energy levels may be at their lowest, restorative yoga poses can be particularly beneficial. Gentle postures such as Supported Child's Pose, Reclining Bound Angle Pose, and Legs-Up-The-Wall encourage relaxation and help alleviate discomfort. Focusing on deep breathing and mindfulness during these poses also aids in reducing stress, which is crucial as stress hormones can exacerbate menstrual symptoms.

As you transition into the follicular phase, energy levels typically rise. This is an excellent time to engage in more dynamic and invigorating yoga sequences. Poses that promote strength and flexibility, such as Warrior II, Triangle Pose, and Sun Salutations, can be integrated to harness the body's growing vitality. This phase is also ideal for incorporating breathwork, or pranayama, techniques that enhance focus and invigorate the body, preparing it for the ovulatory phase.

The ovulatory phase, characterized by peak fertility and often the highest energy levels, allows for the exploration of more challenging poses and peak expressions. Balancing poses like Half Moon Pose or inversions such as Headstand can be practiced to take advantage of the body's full potential during this time. These poses not only build physical strength but also foster a sense of inner confidence and outward expressiveness.

Finally, during the luteal phase, energy may begin to wane as the body prepares for the possibility of pregnancy or the onset of menstruation. This is a period to honor the body's need for slowing down. Transitioning to a gentler practice focusing on hip-opening poses like Pigeon Pose and grounding postures such as Wide-Legged Forward Bend can support the body's natural processes. Additionally, incorporating cooling pranayama techniques can help soothe any premenstrual tension.

Incorporating yoga into cycle alignment is not merely about selecting appropriate poses for each phase but cultivating an intimate dialogue with your body. It requires attentiveness to your body's signals and a willingness to adapt one's practice to the ebb and flow of hormonal changes. By doing so, yoga becomes more than a physical exercise; it transforms into a holistic practice that nurtures the cyclical nature of the female body.

As we delve deeper into the holistic approaches to cycle syncing, it becomes evident that the interplay between various lifestyle factors is key to achieving hormonal harmony. The subsequent discussion will explore another pivotal aspect of this equilibrium: the role of sleep in hormonal balance. By understanding how sleep patterns can be optimized to support the menstrual cycle, you can further enhance your cycle synchronization efforts, leading to a more profound sense of health and vitality.

The Role of Sleep in Hormonal Balance

In the pursuit of achieving hormonal harmony, the significance of sleep cannot be overstated. As we delve into the intricacies of cycle alignment, it becomes clear that the quality and quantity of our slumber play a pivotal role in regulating our endocrine system. The circadian rhythm, an internal clock governing the sleep-wake cycle, is deeply intertwined with the ebb and flow of hormonal levels throughout the menstrual cycle.

The menstrual cycle is a complex interplay of hormones, primarily estrogen and progesterone, which fluctuate naturally. These fluctuations can influence sleep patterns, and conversely, sleep can affect the balance of these hormones. During the follicular phase, rising estrogen levels promote more restful sleep. In contrast, the luteal phase, characterized by higher progesterone levels, may disrupt sleep or lead to fatigue during the day.

Understanding this bidirectional relationship offers a powerful tool for women seeking to align their lifestyles with their biological rhythms. One can foster an environment conducive to hormonal equilibrium by prioritizing sleep hygiene. This involves establishing a consistent sleep schedule, optimizing the sleep environment for comfort and tranquility, and engaging in relaxing pre-sleep routines.

Moreover, the quality of sleep is just as important as its duration. Deep sleep stages are particularly restorative for the body and mind, allowing for the repair of tissues and the consolidation of memories. These stages also contribute to the regulation of cortisol, the stress hormone, which, when imbalanced, can have a cascading effect on other hormones.

To enhance sleep quality, limiting exposure to blue light from screens before bedtime is advisable, as it can interfere with the production of melatonin, the hormone responsible for inducing sleep. Additionally, dietary choices can have an impact; for instance, consuming caffeine or heavy meals too close to bedtime may hinder the ability to fall asleep or stay asleep.

Consider tailoring your evening activities and sleep environment to your menstrual cycle phase. For example, during the luteal phase, when sleep disturbances are more common, it may be beneficial to incorporate relaxation techniques such as meditation or gentle stretching before bed to promote better sleep quality.

By integrating sleep into the broader framework of cycle alignment, you can take proactive steps toward nurturing your hormonal health. This holistic approach enhances overall well-being and empowers you to live in greater synchrony with your body's natural rhythms. Through the strategic alignment of lifestyle choices with the menstrual cycle, you can unlock the full potential of your physical and emotional health, paving the way for a more balanced and fulfilling life.

Chapter Summary

- Mindfulness and meditation are key practices for syncing with the body's natural menstrual cycle, enhancing self-awareness and connection to the body's rhythms.

- Mindfulness involves being present and aware of bodily signals and changes during the menstrual cycle, while meditation can be tailored to the energy levels of each phase.
- These practices can help manage physical symptoms, reduce stress, and promote emotional well-being, leading to more balanced cycles.
- Simple mindfulness exercises like breath awareness or body scans can be incorporated daily, and meditation can start with short sessions focusing on themes relevant to the menstrual phase.
- Herbal remedies have been used for centuries to support menstrual health, with specific herbs beneficial for different phases of the menstrual cycle.
- Consulting with healthcare providers is crucial before using herbal remedies to ensure they are appropriate and to avoid interactions with other medications.
- Acupuncture and Traditional Chinese Medicine offer a holistic approach to cycle syncing, with acupuncture points targeted to balance the body's energy and support menstrual health.
- Yoga practices can be adapted to the menstrual cycle's phases, using restorative poses during menstruation and more active poses during other phases to support hormonal balance and well-being.
- Sleep plays a critical role in hormonal balance, with sleep patterns and menstrual cycle hormones influencing each other.
- Good sleep hygiene and understanding the relationship between sleep and hormonal fluctuations can help align lifestyle with biological rhythms for better health.

9

CREATING YOUR PERSONAL CYCLE ALIGNMENT PLAN

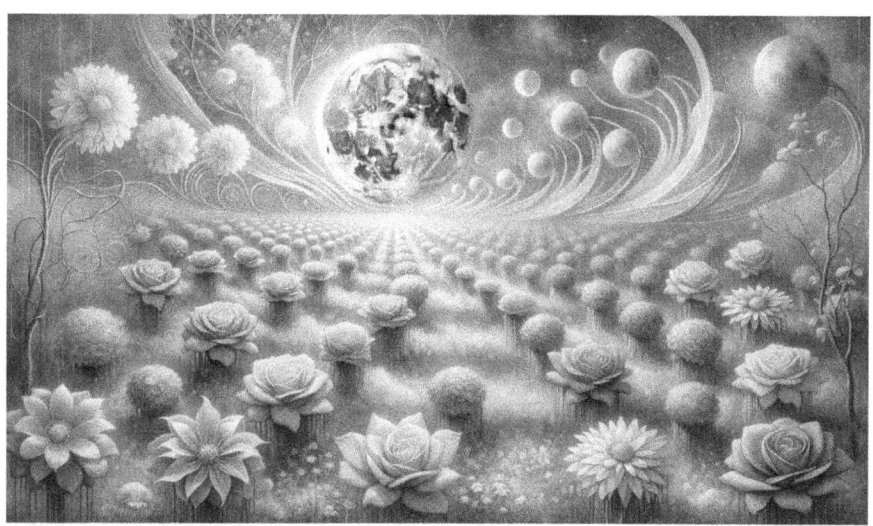

Embarking on the journey of cycle alignment requires a thoughtful assessment of your current lifestyle and menstrual cycle. This process is not about judgment or criticism; it's about understanding your unique rhythms and how they interact with your daily life. By evaluating your current situation, you can create a personalized plan that aligns with your body's natural cycles and supports your overall well-being.

Begin by tracking your menstrual cycle if you haven't already. This is the cornerstone of cycle syncing. Note your period's start and end dates, any symptoms you experience, and how you feel emotionally and physically throughout the different phases.

Next, take a candid look at your current lifestyle. How do your daily activities, work demands, social engagements, and exercise routines align with the different phases of your cycle? Are there times when you feel in sync with your body's needs and times when you don't? For instance, you might notice that high-intensity workouts feel more challenging during your menstrual phase or that you're more sociable and articulate during your ovulatory phase.

Consider also your nutrition. Are you fueling your body with the nutrients it needs to thrive throughout each phase of your cycle? Different phases may benefit from different dietary focuses, such as iron-rich foods during menstruation or more carbohydrates during the luteal phase to support energy levels.

Sleep patterns are another critical aspect to assess. Hormonal shifts throughout your cycle can impact your sleep quality and needs. Pay attention to any changes in your sleep patterns and how they correlate with the different phases of your cycle.

Stress levels and how you manage them should also be evaluated. Chronic stress can disrupt hormonal balance and affect your menstrual cycle. Reflect on the stressors in your life and how you might better manage them to support your hormonal health.

By conducting this comprehensive assessment, you are laying the groundwork for a cycle syncing plan tailored to your body's needs. This personalized approach will help you feel more in tune with your natural rhythms and empower you to make choices that enhance your health and vitality.

With this understanding of your current lifestyle and cycle, you are now ready to set goals and intentions to guide you in making the most of each phase of your cycle. This proactive step will ensure that your cycle syncing plan is well-informed and purpose-driven, setting you up for success in harmonizing your lifestyle with your body's innate patterns.

Setting Goals and Intentions

Embarking on the journey of cycle alignment is akin to setting sail on a voyage of self-discovery and holistic well-being. As you stand at the helm, ready to navigate the waters of your menstrual cycle with newfound knowledge and awareness, it is essential to chart a course that resonates with your aspirations and life circumstances. This voyage begins with setting goals and intentions, which will serve as your guiding stars throughout this transformative process.

Goals and intentions are more than mere wishes; they are the seeds from which the fruits of your efforts will grow. To set them effectively, you must reflect on what you hope to achieve through cycle syncing. You may seek to alleviate physical discomfort, enhance your emotional well-being, or optimize your productivity and creativity. Maybe you aim to deepen your connection with your body's natural rhythms or foster balance and harmony in your daily life. Whatever your desires may be, it is important to articulate them clearly and ensure they align with your core values and lifestyle.

When setting your goals, specificity is your ally. Rather than vague aspirations, define concrete objectives that can be measured and tracked. For instance, if your goal is to reduce premenstrual syndrome (PMS) symptoms, identify which symptoms you wish to address and what improvement would look like. If enhancing your productivity is your aim, determine what that means in the context of your work or personal projects. By being specific, you create a tangible target to aim for, making it easier to recognize progress and maintain motivation.

In addition to setting goals, it is equally important to establish intentions. While goals are the destinations you strive to reach, intentions are the attitudes and mindsets with which you approach your journey. They are the compass that keeps you oriented towards your true north, even when the seas become rough. Intentions could include cultivating patience with your body's processes, practicing self-compassion, or maintaining a sense of curiosity and openness to learning.

As you set your intentions, consider the following questions: How do you want to feel throughout your cycle? What personal strengths can you draw upon to support your goals? What mindset shifts might be necessary to embrace the ebbs and flows of your cycle? By answering these questions, you can craft intentions that not only complement your goals but also empower you to approach each phase of your cycle with grace and resilience.

Remember, setting goals and intentions is not a one-time event but an ongoing dialogue with yourself. As you progress in your cycle alignment journey, revisit and refine your goals and intentions to reflect your growth and any new insights you gain. This iterative process ensures that your cycle alignment plan remains dynamic and responsive to your evolving needs.

With your goals and intentions now clearly defined, you are well-prepared to move forward with designing your personalized cycle alignment strategy. This strategy will be your roadmap, detailing the practical steps you will take to align your daily life with the natural rhythms of your menstrual cycle. Here, the seeds of your goals and intentions will take root, and with careful nurturing, they will grow into a life that is in harmonious sync with your body's innate wisdom.

Designing Your Personalized Cycle Alignment Strategy

With your goals and intentions clearly outlined, it's time to move forward into the heart of cycle synchronization: designing your personalized strategy. This process is akin to crafting a tailored wellness plan that aligns with the unique rhythms of your body. It's about creating harmony between your lifestyle and your menstrual cycle, allowing you to harness the ebb and flow of your hormonal landscape.

Let's focus on the four distinct phases of your menstrual cycle: the menstrual phase, the follicular phase, the ovulatory phase, and the luteal phase. Each of these phases comes with its own hormonal fluctuations that can influence your energy levels, mood, and overall well-being. Understanding these phases is the foundation upon which you will build your cycle-syncing strategy. Here's a summary of some of the strategies we covered in previous chapters:

- **Menstrual Phase:** During this time, when your energy may be at its lowest, consider gentle activities such as yoga, meditation, or light walking. Nutritionally, support your body with warm, nourishing foods rich in iron and protein to replenish what is lost during menstruation.
- **Follicular Phase:** As your energy rises, this is an opportune time to tackle new projects and engage in more vigorous exercise. Your diet can shift to include more raw foods and lighter fare that align with your body's increasing momentum.
- **Ovulatory Phase:** With energy typically at its peak, capitalize on this by scheduling important meetings or social engagements. High-impact workouts can be most beneficial during this phase. Foods rich in fiber can help support the body's natural detoxification processes.
- **Luteal Phase:** As you wind down, it's vital to start slowing your pace. Focus on completing tasks rather than starting new ones. Gentle exercise like swimming or cycling can be soothing. Cravings might arise; balance them with healthy fats and complex carbohydrates to maintain stable blood sugar levels.

Now, let's consider the personalization of your strategy. Start by tracking your cycle, if you aren't already, to pinpoint the length and particularities of each phase for you. This isn't a one-size-fits-all approach; your cycle is unique, and your plan should reflect that.

Next, integrate your goals and intentions. If you aim for improved fitness, align your workout intensity with the natural fluctuations in your energy. For career-focused goals, schedule demanding tasks during your follicular and ovulatory phases when you're likely to feel more outgoing and assertive.

Remember, this strategy should enhance your life, not complicate it. Flexibility is key. If a high-energy activity is planned, but you're not feeling up to it, it's okay to adjust. Listening to your body is paramount; the goal is to sync with your cycle, not to be ruled by it.

As you design your plan, consider all aspects of your life—work, relationships, personal growth, and rest. Each should ebb and flow with your cycle, allowing you to optimize your time and energy effectively.

In the next section, we'll delve into implementing your plan, ensuring it fits seamlessly into your lifestyle, and making adjustments as needed. Remember, cycle syncing is a dynamic process, and your strategy should evolve with you as you gain insights and experience with your body's rhythms.

Implementing and Adjusting Your Plan

Having designed your personalized cycle syncing strategy, you are poised to embark on a transformative journey. Implementing your plan is a dynamic process that requires patience, observation, and the willingness to adapt. As you step into this phase, remember that your body's responses are unique, and your plan should be as fluid as the cycles you aim to sync with.

Begin by integrating the elements of your cycle-syncing strategy into your daily routine. This might involve adjusting your diet, exercise regimen, social engagements, and work tasks to align with the different phases of your menstrual cycle. For instance, when energy levels typically rise during the follicular phase, you might schedule more demanding projects or start new initiatives. Conversely, during the luteal phase, when you feel more introspective, you could plan for tasks requiring less social interaction and more detail-oriented work.

As you implement these changes, it's crucial to maintain a non-judgmental attitude towards yourself. Some days will be easier than others, and that's perfectly normal. The goal is not to achieve perfection but to cultivate a deeper understanding and harmony with your body's natural rhythms.

Monitoring your body's reactions to these adjustments is vital. You may find that certain assumptions you made during the planning stage don't hold true in practice. Perhaps a particular type of exercise you thought would be energizing during one phase of your cycle leaves you feeling depleted. Or you may discover that you're more social during the luteal phase than anticipated. These insights are valuable and should be used to refine your plan.

Adjusting your plan is not a sign of failure; it is a sign of attunement. It means you are listening to your body and respecting its signals. Make small, incremental changes rather than sweeping overhauls to avoid overwhelming yourself and observe the effect of each adjustment better.

Remember, the ultimate aim of cycle synchronization is to enhance your well-being and empower you to live in sync with your body's natural rhythms. This process is inherently personal and will evolve over time. Embrace the learning curve and allow your cycle alignment plan to be a living document that grows and changes as you do.

As you continue implementing and adjusting your plan, you'll gather valuable data about your body and its cycles. This data will be the foundation for the next step in your journey: tracking progress and making data-driven decisions, which will further refine your approach to cycle syncing and help you achieve the balance and harmony you seek.

Tracking Progress and Making Data-Driven Decisions

Remember to recognize that this is not a static plan but a dynamic process that evolves with you. The key to harnessing the full potential of cycle alignment lies in meticulously tracking your progress and making informed decisions based on the data you collect. This approach ensures that your personal cycle alignment plan is not only tailored to your unique rhythms but also adaptable to the changes your body may experience over time.

Begin by establishing a baseline. Document your physical, emotional, and mental states daily. Note your energy levels, mood fluctuations, sleep quality, dietary cravings, and physical symptoms. Utilize a journal or a digital tracking tool designed for cycle syncing to streamline this process. The objective is to gather enough data to discern patterns that correlate with the different phases of your menstrual cycle.

As you collect data, you'll start to notice trends. You may see that your energy peaks during the ovulatory phase or requires more rest during the luteal phase. These insights are invaluable as they guide you in fine-tuning your cycle syncing plan. For instance, you may schedule demanding tasks when your energy is naturally higher or incorporate more self-care practices when you need additional rest.

Pay attention to the outliers – days when you don't feel as expected based on your cycle phase. These instances can be just as informative, prompting you to consider external factors such as stress, diet, or exercise that may influence your well-being. Acknowledging these variables allows you to adjust your plan to support your body's needs better.

Remember, tracking aims not to judge or critique your experiences but to understand them. This understanding empowers you to make data-driven decisions that enhance your well-being. For example, if you consistently notice digestive discomfort during a specific phase, you might experiment with dietary adjustments. Or, if your creativity surges in the follicular phase, you could align your work on creative projects to this period for maximum efficacy.

Regularly review your tracking data – a monthly check-in is a good practice. Assess what's working and what isn't. Celebrate the successes, no matter how small, and consider what adjustments could be made to address any challenges. This is not a one-time evaluation but a continuous process that echoes the cyclical nature of your body.

Lastly, be patient with yourself. Cycle alignment is a personal journey, and it may take several cycles to fully understand and harmonize with your body's rhythms. Each cycle is an opportunity to learn more about yourself and to refine your approach. Trust in the process, and allow your personal cycle syncing plan to be a living document that grows and changes as you do.

By embracing a systematic and data-driven approach to tracking your progress, you are equipping yourself with the knowledge and flexibility needed to create a cycle-syncing plan that genuinely resonates with your body's innate wisdom. This is not just a plan but a pathway to a more attuned and empowered you.

Chapter Summary

- Begin by tracking your menstrual cycle phases: menstrual, follicular, ovulatory, and luteal, noting symptoms and emotional and physical states in each phase.
- Assess how your current lifestyle, including activities, work, social life, and exercise, aligns with your cycle phases.
- Evaluate your nutrition, ensuring you consume phase-appropriate foods that support your hormonal fluctuations.
- Monitor sleep patterns and their correlation with your cycle, as hormonal shifts can affect sleep quality.
- Reflect on stress levels and management techniques, considering the impact of stress on hormonal balance.
- Set specific, measurable goals and intentions for cycle synchronization, aligned with personal values and aspirations.
- Design a personalized cycle alignment strategy, adjusting activities, diet, and tasks to each cycle phase.
- Implement and adjust your plan based on body responses, maintaining flexibility and a non-judgmental attitude towards yourself.

10

THE FUTURE OF CYCLE ALIGNMENT

As we delve into the realm of cycle alignment, it is essential to recognize that this field is not static but dynamic and burgeoning with potential. The concept of cycle alignment has gained traction in recent years. However, the future holds even more promise as emerging research and developments unfold, offering deeper insights and more refined approaches to this personalized health strategy.

One of the most exciting areas of development is the increasing understanding of the molecular and physiological mechanisms behind the menstrual cycle. Scientists are beginning to unravel the complex interplay of hormones, such as estrogen and progesterone, and their systemic effects on the body. This research not only reveals why specific symptoms manifest during different phases of the cycle but also how we might mitigate them effectively. For example, studies are exploring how fluctuations in hormone levels influence mood, energy, metabolism, and even the microbiome, which could lead to more nuanced cycle-syncing protocols.

Another promising avenue of research is investigating the impact of cycle syncing on various health conditions. Preliminary studies suggest that aligning lifestyle choices with hormonal fluctuations could potentially alleviate symptoms of conditions like polycystic ovary syndrome, endometriosis, and premenstrual syndrom. As research progresses, cycle synchronization could become a cornerstone of treatment plans for these and other hormone-related disorders.

The potential of cycle synchronization extends beyond symptom management. There is a growing body of evidence to suggest that it could play a role in enhancing overall well-being and performance. For example, by syncing exercise routines with the menstrual cycle, women may optimize their workouts, improve recovery, and even prevent injuries. Similarly, aligning nutrition with hormonal changes could maximize nutrient absorption and support metabolic health.

The implications of these developments are vast. As we gain a more sophisticated understanding of the menstrual cycle's influence on the body, cycle alignment could evolve into a highly personalized form of health optimization. It could empower individuals to manage symptoms and enhance their physical and mental performance, tailor their nutrition, and even improve their long-term health outcomes.

In the future, we may see the development of comprehensive cycle alignment programs that are as commonplace as general dietary and fitness plans are today. These programs would be backed by robust scientific research and could be tailored to each individual's unique hormonal profile, lifestyle, and health goals.

As we stand on the cusp of these advancements, it is clear that the future of cycle synchronization is bright. With continued research and development, this approach has the potential to transform the way women live in harmony with their bodies, unlocking a new paradigm of personalized health and wellness.

The Role of Technology in Cycle Alignment

As we delve into the transformative potential of technology in cycle alignment, it is essential to recognize its profound impact on personal health management. The advent of sophisticated apps and wearable devices has revolutionized the way individuals can monitor and understand their menstrual cycles, offering a personalized approach to health that was once unattainable.

Integrating technology into cycle alignment is not merely a matter of convenience but a profound expansion of personal agency and self-knowledge. Women and individuals with menstrual cycles are now equipped with tools that provide insights into their hormonal fluctuations, fertility windows, and potential health issues. These technological advancements can demystify the menstrual cycle, transforming it from a taboo subject into a wellspring of valuable health data.

Wearable technology, in particular, has taken the forefront in this revolution. Devices that track physiological parameters such as body temperature, heart rate, and sleep patterns are becoming increasingly sophisticated. They offer real-time data that can help predict energy levels, mood changes, and nutritional needs when correlated with menstrual cycle phases. This level of detail empowers individuals to make informed decisions about exercise, diet, social engagements, and work productivity, all tailored to the rhythm of their cycles.

Moreover, the data collected by these technologies is not only beneficial on an individual level but also has the potential to contribute to a larger pool of research. With user consent, anonymized health data can be invaluable for scientific studies, leading to a deeper understanding of menstrual health and its connection to overall well-being. This collective knowledge could drive the development of more effective treatments for menstrual-related disorders and pave the way for a future where cycle alignment is not an alternative method but a standard practice in personalized healthcare.

The role of artificial intelligence (AI) in this domain cannot be overstated. AI algorithms are becoming increasingly adept at pattern recognition, learning from the menstrual cycle data input by users to provide more accurate predictions and personalized health insights. This could lead to AI-powered virtual health assistants that track and analyze cycle data and offer recommendations for optimizing physical and mental health based on an individual's unique cycle patterns.

However, with the rise of technology comes the imperative responsibility to address privacy concerns. The intimate nature of menstrual health data necessitates stringent security measures to protect user information. Developers and companies behind cycle alignment technologies must prioritize data encryption and ethical data usage policies to maintain trust and ensure that users' personal health information is safeguarded against unauthorized access.

In conclusion, the role of technology in cycle alignment is a testament to the remarkable strides made in personal health management. By harnessing the power of wearable devices, apps, and AI, individuals gain unprecedented control over their health and well-being. As we continue to explore these technologies' capabilities, we must advocate for responsible data practices and continue to educate on the importance of menstrual health, ensuring that the future of cycle alignment is not only technologically advanced but also inclusive, secure, and empowering.

Expanding the Conversation: Education and Advocacy

In pursuing a future where cycle alignment is not only a well-understood concept but also a widely accepted practice, the expansion of conversation through education and advocacy is a pivotal step. This expansion is not merely about spreading awareness; it is about embedding the knowledge of menstrual health and cycle alignment into the fabric of society, thereby empowering individuals to make informed decisions about their bodies and overall well-being.

Education, in this context, takes on a multi-faceted approach. It begins in the classroom, where comprehensive sex education should include detailed information on menstrual cycles and the impact they have on an individual's physical and emotional state. By introducing cycle alignment as a topic of study, educators can provide young people with the tools to understand and work with their bodies rather than against them. When imparted early, this knowledge can lay the groundwork for a lifetime of informed health choices and self-awareness.

Beyond the classroom, education must also permeate into the healthcare system. From general practitioners to specialists, medical professionals should be equipped with the latest research and understanding of cycle alignment. This ensures that when patients come with questions or seek advice on menstrual health, they receive guidance that is not only empathetic but also scientifically sound and tailored to their unique rhythms.

Advocacy is crucial in normalizing the conversation around menstrual health and cycle syncing. Advocates can work to dismantle the taboos and stigmas that have long shrouded discussions of menstruation. Advocates can foster a culture of openness and acceptance by creating platforms where individuals feel safe and supported in sharing their experiences. This, in turn, can influence policy-making, leading to menstrual health considerations in the workplace, such as flexible scheduling and environments that accommodate the varying phases of the menstrual cycle.

Moreover, advocacy efforts can help to secure funding for further research into cycle alignment. With a robust body of evidence, the potential benefits of cycle syncing can be more widely recognized, leading to its integration into health and wellness programs. This could pave the way for apps and technology, discussed in the previous section, to be more than just personal tools; they could become part of a more significant, systemic approach to health management.

Expanding the conversation through education and advocacy is about creating a world where cycle syncing is not an esoteric concept but a common practice. It is about ensuring that everyone has the knowledge and support to harness the power of their menstrual cycle, leading to a future where cycle alignment is as routine as any other aspect of health and wellness.

Building a Community Around Menstrual Health

In the pursuit of a future where cycle synchronization is not only understood but also embraced, the creation of a robust community around menstrual health stands as a pivotal step. This community, envisioned as a collective of individuals from diverse backgrounds, would serve as a sanctuary for sharing experiences, offering support, and disseminating knowledge about the intricacies of menstrual cycles and the broader implications of hormonal health.

The foundation of such a community is rooted in the recognition that menstrual health is not a niche concern but a universal aspect of human biology that affects half of the population directly and the other half indirectly. By fostering open dialogue and creating safe spaces, both virtual and physical, individuals can learn from one another, share their triumphs and challenges, and normalize the conversation around menstruation and cycle alignment.

To build this community, a multi-faceted approach is necessary. Firstly, leveraging technology to connect individuals across geographical boundaries can provide a platform for those seeking guidance and camaraderie. Online forums, social media groups, and dedicated apps can offer resources and facilitate discussions that empower individuals to take charge of their menstrual health through cycle alignment.

Secondly, local meet-ups and workshops can complement online interactions, providing a tangible sense of community. These gatherings can range from educational seminars led by healthcare professionals to informal support groups. By meeting face-to-face, individuals can form stronger bonds and a sense of belonging, essential for sustaining engagement and fostering a supportive network.

Furthermore, collaboration with healthcare providers is crucial. By involving experts in the field, the community can ensure that the information shared is accurate and up-to-date. Healthcare professionals can also benefit from such a community by gaining insights into the real-world experiences of those they treat, leading to more empathetic and personalized care.

In addition to these efforts, the community must be inclusive and acknowledge the diversity of experiences with menstrual health. Recognizing that menstrual cycles and hormonal changes affect everyone differently, the community should celebrate this diversity and strive to cater to various needs and perspectives. This inclusivity extends to individuals with various health conditions, gender identities, and cultural backgrounds, all of whom should find their place within the community.

Lastly, the community should not only be a source of support but also a force for change. By uniting individuals who are informed and passionate about menstrual health, the community can advocate for better resources, research, and recognition of the importance of cycle syncing in public health agendas.

In essence, building a community around menstrual health is about creating a movement that champions the well-being of individuals through shared knowledge, mutual support, and collective action. Through this community, the future of cycle alignment can be realized, ensuring that every individual can live in harmony with their body's natural rhythms.

Envisioning a Society in Sync with Cycles

In the tapestry of human health and well-being, menstrual health has often been a thread that's been overlooked or hidden away. However, as we look to the future, we can envision a society that not only acknowledges but also embraces the concept of cycle alignment. This is a future where the natural rhythms of the menstrual cycle are harmoniously integrated into the fabric of daily life, fostering an environment that supports the physical, emotional, and mental health of those who menstruate.

Imagine a world where workplaces, educational institutions, and social settings are all tuned to the menstrual cycle. In this society, the stigma surrounding menstruation dissipates, replaced by a culture of openness and understanding. Work schedules and academic deadlines could be more flexible, accommodating the varying energy levels and cognitive states associated with the different phases of the menstrual cycle. This would not only enhance productivity but also promote a sense of well-being and respect for the body's natural processes.

In such a society, menstrual health education is comprehensive and begins early. Both young people and adults are equipped with the knowledge to understand and work with their cycles rather than against them.

This education extends beyond biological aspects, encompassing the emotional and psychological influences of hormonal fluctuations. With this knowledge, individuals can make informed decisions about diet, exercise, social engagements, and work tasks that align with their cycle phases.

Healthcare systems in this envisioned future are more responsive and personalized. Medical professionals are trained in cycle alignment, enabling them to provide care tailored to the individual's cycle phase. This could lead to more effective treatments for menstrual-related disorders and a greater emphasis on preventative care. Technology, too, plays a pivotal role, with apps and devices designed to track and analyze menstrual cycles, offering insights and recommendations for optimal living in accordance with one's cycle.

In the realm of personal relationships, cycle alignment fosters empathy and communication. Partners and family members are more attuned to the needs and experiences of those who menstruate, leading to stronger, more supportive bonds. Social plans can be made with consideration of one's cycle, ensuring that activities are aligned with the energy and mood of the individual.

Furthermore, the future of cycle alignment extends to public policy. Governments and institutions could implement policies supporting menstrual health, such as providing menstrual products in public restrooms and ensuring access to health education and care. These policies would not only support those who menstruate but also signal a broader commitment to public health and gender equality.

In this future, cycle alignment is not a niche concept but a widespread practice that enhances the quality of life. It is a testament to a society that values the health and well-being of all its members, recognizing the profound impact that syncing with natural cycles can have on individual and collective prosperity.

As we move forward, the potential of cycle alignment is boundless. It offers a pathway to a more attuned, empathetic, and health-conscious society. By embracing the natural rhythms of the menstrual cycle, we can create a future that is not only in sync with our bodies but also with our potential for growth and harmony.

Chapter Summary

- The future of cycle synchronization is promising, with ongoing research into how diet, exercise, and lifestyle can be tailored to the menstrual cycle phases.
- Scientists are uncovering how hormonal fluctuations affect mood, energy, metabolism, and the microbiome, which may lead to more effective cycle alignment methods.
- Preliminary studies indicate that cycle syncing could help alleviate symptoms of hormonal disorders like PCOS, endometriosis, and PMS.
- Cycle alignment may enhance overall well-being and performance, optimizing workouts, recovery, and nutrient absorption based on menstrual cycle phases.
- Technology, including apps and wearable devices, is revolutionizing cycle alignment by providing personalized menstrual cycle data and health insights.
- Artificial intelligence could further personalize health recommendations based on menstrual cycle patterns, but privacy and data security are paramount concerns.
- Education and advocacy are key to normalizing cycle alignment, with a need for comprehensive menstrual health education and informed healthcare professionals.
- Building a community around menstrual health can offer support, share knowledge, and advocate for public health policies that recognize the importance and benefits of cycle alignment.

YOUR JOURNEY BEYOND THE PAGES

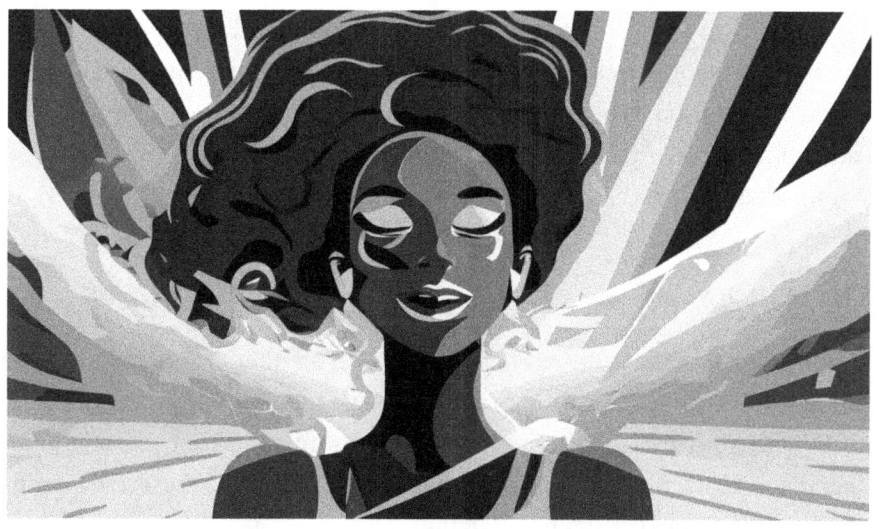

As we reach the concluding chapter of this book, it's time to pause and reflect on what you've learned and how far you've come. Think back to the beginning of this book and consider the changes in how you now understand and relate to your cycle. This reflection is crucial in solidifying the knowledge and practices you've acquired.

Take a moment to appreciate the growth in your self-awareness and the proactive steps you've taken to align your daily life with your cycle's rhythm. Whether you've made dietary adjustments, modified your exercise routine, or found new ways to manage stress, each change contributes to a healthier, more balanced you.

Use journaling or quiet contemplation to process your journey. Consider which chapters resonated the most and why. Reflect on how your perspective on your cycle has shifted and what this means for your future.

Acknowledging your journey is also about recognizing that learning and growth are ongoing processes. There may have been challenges along the way, but each one has offered valuable lessons and opportunities for personal development.

As you close this book, remember that the end of this reading is just the beginning of a lifelong practice. Keep revisiting these pages and your reflections as you evolve and deepen your connection with your cycle. Your journey with your body's natural rhythms doesn't stop here—it's a continuous path of discovery and empowerment.

Celebrating Your Wins

Remember to take a moment every now and then to celebrate your achievements. Recognize the progress you've made in aligning your lifestyle with your cycle. Whether it's feeling more energized, experiencing less discomfort, or finding greater balance in your life, these are significant milestones worth acknowledging.

Celebrate the small victories as well as the big ones. You may have started to notice patterns in your energy levels and have used this knowledge to plan your activities more effectively. Or perhaps you've found that certain foods help you feel better at different times of the month. No matter how minor they seem, these insights and changes are steps towards a more harmonious life.

Sharing your successes can be incredibly powerful. It not only reinforces your achievements but also encourages others to explore their paths to cycle alignment. Whether you share with friends, family, or a wider audience, your story can inspire and guide.

Creating a personal ritual to celebrate these wins can also be beneficial. It could be as simple as taking a moment at the end of each cycle to reflect on what went well or treating yourself to something special as a reward for your efforts. This act of celebration helps to solidify the positive changes you've made.

Remember, regardless of size, each win is a step forward in your journey. These accomplishments are the results and motivators that propel you toward continued growth and well-being. So, take the time to honor your hard work and the positive outcomes that have come from it. Your journey doesn't end here; each cycle brings new opportunities to build on these successes and continue to thrive.

Overcoming Challenges

As we draw the final threads of our narrative together, it's essential to acknowledge that aligning with your cycle is not without its hurdles. You may have encountered obstacles along the way, or perhaps you're still navigating through them. It's essential to recognize that these challenges are a natural part of the journey, and overcoming them is a testament to your resilience.

Remember, the road to harmony with your cycle is much like the cycle itself—dynamic and ever-changing. There will be days when everything falls into place effortlessly and others when it feels like an uphill climb. During these times, your strength and determination are truly tested, and it's also when the most profound growth can occur.

If you've faced setbacks, take a moment to reflect on what they've taught you. Each challenge is an opportunity to learn more about your body and yourself. They prompt you to adapt, to seek out new strategies, and to reach out for support when needed. Embrace these lessons, for they are valuable guides on your path forward.

Lean on the community of fellow cycle explorers you've met along the way, whether in person or through the vast connections of the online world. There is strength in numbers, and the shared wisdom of others can provide comfort and practical advice as you continue to navigate your journey.

As you move beyond this book, carry with you the understanding that challenges are not roadblocks but stepping stones to greater self-awareness and empowerment. With each obstacle you overcome, you pave the way for a smoother journey ahead for yourself and others who walk the path beside you.

So, as we close this chapter, remember that the true essence of overcoming is not in never facing difficulties but rising each time we fall. Your journey with your cycle is a continuous evolution, where each challenge surmounted adds a new layer of strength to your story. Keep this spirit of perseverance close to your heart, and step forward with confidence, knowing that you are equipped to meet and master whatever lies ahead.

Continuing the Cycle Alignment Journey

As we approach the end of this written voyage, remember that the true journey doesn't have a final destination. The practice of aligning with your cycle is an ongoing adventure that continues to unfold each month. It's a lifelong commitment to listening to your body and responding to its needs with care and understanding.

Maintaining the harmony between your lifestyle and your cycle requires consistent attention and nurturing. It's like tending to a garden; regular care ensures it flourishes. Keep the principles you've learned in this book close to your heart, and integrate them into the fabric of your daily life. Let them become as natural to you as breathing.

Staying motivated can be challenging, but remember why you started this journey. Revisit your reflections and celebrate your wins to remind yourself of the positive changes you've experienced. This is the fuel that will keep your inner fire burning brightly.

As you move forward, continue to explore and deepen your understanding of your body. Stay curious and open to new research, insights, and strategies that can enhance your cycle alignment practice. Knowledge is a powerful tool, and there's always more to learn.

Encourage yourself to be flexible and adaptable. As your life changes, so may your cycle and how you align with it. Embrace these changes as part of life's natural ebb and flow, and adjust your practices accordingly.

Remember, this book is a starting point, a foundation upon which you can build a more prosperous, more attuned relationship with your cycle. Keep it as a trusted guide, but also trust in your wisdom and the wisdom of your body. You have all the tools you need to continue this journey with confidence and grace.

So, as we part ways in text, know that your cycle alignment journey is just beginning. Carry forward the lessons, the love, and the commitment to your well-being that you've cultivated here. Your path ahead is bright with the promise of continued growth, balance, and empowerment.

Looking Forward

Now, let's cast our gaze forward to the horizon of your journey. The chapters behind us have been a map to guide you, but the path ahead is yours to forge with the wisdom and understanding you've gained. The future of aligning with your cycle is a canvas stretched out before you, ready for your continued exploration and growth.

Envision a world where the knowledge you now hold is shared and celebrated—a world where the cycles of our bodies are honored as a source of insight and strength. You are now a beacon in this movement, a pioneer in living in harmony with your body's natural rhythms. Embrace this role and consider how you can inspire others to embark on their journeys of discovery and alignment.

The conversation around menstrual health and cycle awareness is ever-evolving; you are part of that evolution. Advocate for this awareness in your circles and help to weave this understanding into the fabric of society. Each voice that joins this chorus amplifies the message, bringing us closer to a future where cycle alignment is not just a personal practice but a collective awakening.

As you close this book, remember that the end of this reading is just one milestone in your lifelong relationship with your cycle. Continue to nurture this relationship, listen, and respond to your body with love and respect. The empowerment you've found within these pages is a flame that will light your way through all the cycles to come.

So, dear reader, as you step beyond the pages of this book, carry with you the courage, the knowledge, and the joy you've discovered. Let them be your companions as you journey forward, creating a life that is not only in sync with your cycle but also in tune with the deepest parts of yourself.

Here's to the future—a future where each of us lives in full bloom, aligned with the powerful rhythms of our bodies, and where every cycle is a celebration of our innate wisdom and beauty.

ABOUT THE AUTHOR

Lila Lacy is a passionate advocate for women's health and well-being. With years of experience working in women's health advocacy, Lila has dedicated her career to empowering women through knowledge and support.

Her journey began with a deep interest in the intricate dance of hormones within the female body and how they influence every aspect of health and daily life. Recognizing the lack of accessible, comprehensive information on the subject, Lila set out to bridge the gap between medical research and the everyday experiences of women.

Lila writes with the conviction that understanding one's body is the first step toward wellness and self-empowerment. Her work is characterized by its empathetic tone, practical advice, and unwavering commitment to debunking myths surrounding women's health.

Lila Lacy continues to be a beacon of hope and a source of cutting-edge information for women seeking to reclaim their health and harmony with their bodies. Her books not only educate but also inspire readers to make lasting changes that resonate through all facets of their lives.

When she's not writing or speaking, Lila enjoys practicing yoga, experimenting with hormone-friendly recipes, and spending time in nature.

www.ingramcontent.com/pod-product-compliance
Lightning Source LLC
Chambersburg PA
CBHW071720020426
42333CB00017B/2341